The Global Vegan Family Cookbook

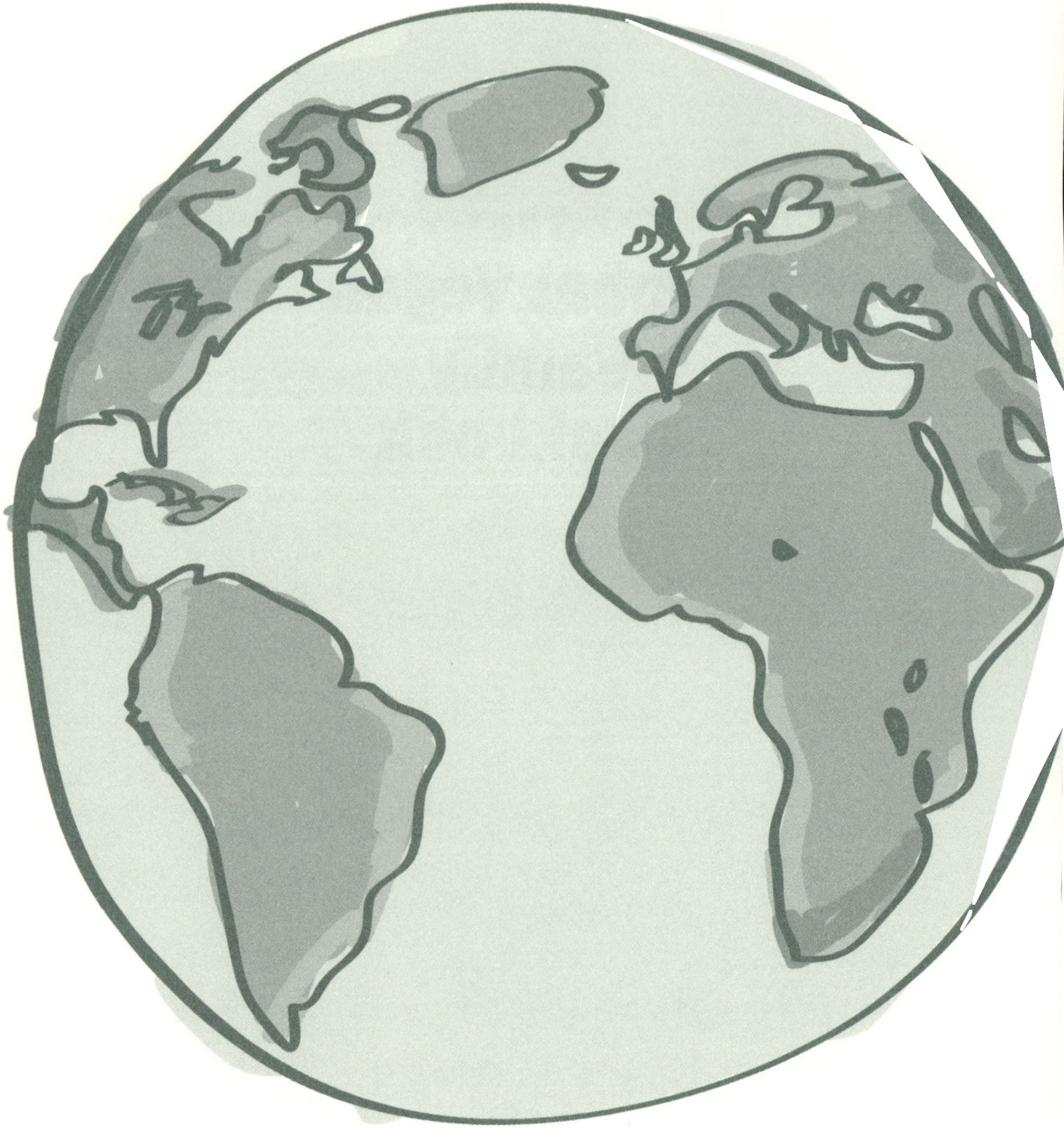

The Global Vegan Family Cookbook

BRIAN P. McCARTHY

LANTERN BOOKS • NEW YORK • A DIVISION OF BOOKLIGHT INC.

2013
Lantern Books
128 Second Place
Brooklyn, NY 11231
www.lanternbooks.com

Printed in the United States of America

Library of Congress Cataloging-in-Publication Data

McCarthy, Brian P., 1965–
The global vegan family cookbook / By Brian P. McCarthy.
pages cm
Includes bibliographical references and index.
ISBN 978-1-59056-415-8 (pbk. : alk. paper) — ISBN 978-1-59056-416-5 (ebook)
1. Vegan cooking. I. Title.
TX837.M466 2012
641.5′636—dc23

2012033487

MIX
Paper from responsible sources
FSC® C011935
www.fsc.org

To my loving wife

who sat next to me many
countless hours, days, weeks, and months
helping me edit recipes.
I could not have done this without you.
You are amazing!

Table of Contents

Welcome!

As the cultures of the world become closer and more familiar to us, we have the opportunity to enjoy international cuisine more easily and more frequently. When I was growing up in Oregon there were perhaps four or five international restaurants in my town. Now four or five international restaurants can be found by biking down just a couple of blocks. Because many cuisines include dishes without meat and dairy by their nature, vegan cuisine has become more widely available. With all of this interesting food being served, I was motivated to learn this fare and share it with others.

But was my international cooking authentic? Would it be accepted by the international community? I put it to the test when I worked at the technology company Intel, serving meals that included Papa Rellenos and Vegetable Vindaloo. My lunch lines started filling with a diverse group which included, among others, Indian, Chinese, Russian, French, Irish, Hungarian, and American employees. With the coaching of my devoted customers, I started serving 80-130 vegan international meals five days a week for the next three years. Over this period of time I learned how to cook international food as efficiently and economically as possible.

Lately I have had the honor to cook at the Massachusetts Institute of Technology (MIT). Cooking vegan food for MIT students is rewarding, to say the least. While they feed their minds, I get to feed their bodies. MIT students are not much different than corporate employees in their diversity (a primary difference is MIT students can come to the cafeteria in their pajamas). The students are very educated, adventuresome, and respectful, and many of them eat vegan or vegetarian.

In this cookbook I've tried to include recipes from every corner of the world, some which you may be familiar with and some that may sound strange (but I hope you'll try anyway). I've included recipes from the United States, since parts of the U.S. are as varied as any country. In particular I've added a couple of desserts from my home state of Oregon. Most of the recipes are for dishes that you would eat if you were in that part of the world, while some are "fusion" dishes from my own repertoire.

Whether these recipes are from far away or closer to home, I hope you find them as useful as I have in helping to bring the members of our world community together.

Appetizers:

Italy

Bruschetta with Roasted Garlic Tapenade

Kalamata olives are named after the Greek city of the same name, which is also known for its dates.

Yield: 14

7 cloves garlic

¼ cup olive oil

1 cup pitted Kalamata olives

¼ cup small, pickled and salted capers, rinsed and drained

1 bunch basil, stems removed

16-oz. baguette

7 cherry tomatoes, cut into sixths

Preheat oven to 375°F.

In a small baking dish, toss garlic with olive oil.

Bake for 20 minutes.

Cool garlic and olive oil for 30 minutes.

In a food processor, process the roasted garlic, olive oil, olives, capers, and basil (reserve some of the small basil leaves for garnish if preferred) until nearly smooth.

Chill.

Slice baguette into 14 diagonal slices and place in single layer on a baking sheet.

Bake until lightly crisp but still slightly tender in the middle, about two minutes. Cool 10 minutes.

Spread a thin layer of tapenade onto each baguette slice and garnish with 3 pieces of tomato and a reserved basil leaf.

Serve immediately or cover and chill until needed (remove from refrigerator 30 minutes before serving).

Italy

Crostini with Sun-dried Tomato Cream Cheese

Crostini means "little toasts" in Italian.

Yield: 14

6 sun-dried tomatoes*

8 oz. vegan cream cheese

½ tsp. salt

16-oz. baguette

3 Tbs. olive oil

15 oz. jar whole pimento stuffed olives, sliced

Preheat oven to 375°F.

Place sun-dried tomatoes* in boiling water and boil until tender, about five minutes. Drain off water.

In a food processor, process the sun-dried tomatoes, cream cheese, and salt until smooth.

Chill cream cheese mixture.

Slice baguette into ½-inch rounds. Place in single layer on a baking sheet. Brush baguette rounds with olive oil.

Bake until lightly crisp, about five minutes. Cool 10 minutes.

Spread a thin layer of the cream cheese mixture on each baguette round and garnish with sliced olives.

Serve immediately or cover and chill until needed (remove from refrigerator 30 minutes before serving).

** Omit this step if using sun-dried tomatoes in oil.*

Cumin Naan with Baba Ganoush

In East India, naan is traditionally baked on the inside walls of high-heat tandoori ovens.

Yield: 8 servings

2½ cups Baba Ganoush (pg. 287)

2 Tbs. sesame seeds

2 tsp. cumin powder

2 tsp. salt

2 Tbs. olive oil

1 Tbs. active dry yeast (¼-oz. package)

1½ cups warm water (110°F)

½ tsp. sugar

3½ cups flour*, divided

* *Use part whole wheat flour if you prefer.*

Prepare Baba Ganoush and chill until needed.

In a small saucepan, combine sesame seeds, cumin powder, salt and oil. Cook on medium heat until bubbly. Set aside.

In a large bowl, whisk together the yeast, water, and sugar. Let sit 10 minutes.

Whisk the seasoned oil mixture into the yeast mixture.

Whisk in one cup of the flour.

Stir in the remaining 2½ cups of flour.

On a floured surface, knead dough for seven minutes.

Place in a large, lightly oiled bowl and cover with clear wrap.

Let rise until doubled in size, about 45 minutes.

Punch down dough and knead for one minute.

Divide dough into eight pieces.

Roll each piece into an 8-inch round.

Preheat griddle to 400°F, or medium heat with a skillet.

Grill on a dry griddle for one minute on each side or until done.

Serve with Baba Ganoush.

Grilled Plantains with Mole Sauce

Plantains are considered a cooking banana and are used much like potatoes. A green plantain will ripen to the yellow state but can take several days.

Yield: 4 servings

1 cup Mole Sauce (pg. 305)

2 cups cold water

2 Tbs. salt

¾ tsp. garlic powder

¾ tsp. onion powder

½ tsp. salt

2 yellow plantain bananas

Vegetable oil for grilling (¼-inch in pan)

Prepare Mole Sauce and set aside.

Whisk together cold water and two Tbs. salt and set aside.

Combine the garlic powder, onion powder and ½ tsp. salt and set aside.

Peel plantains and cut into ½-inch thick diagonal pieces.

Preheat oil in large skillet. Grill plantains with oil until browned, about two minutes on each side.

Place fried plantains in salt water mixture (from step two) for one minute.

Remove plantains and pat dry with paper towels.

On a cutting board and using the palm of your hand, slightly squash plantains to about ¼-inch thick.

In a large skillet, re-grill plantains with oil for an additional two minutes on each side.

Remove plantains from oil and toss with garlic powder, onion powder, and salt mixture.

Serve warm plantains with warm Mole Sauce on the side.

Southern USA

Hush Puppies with Chipotle Dipping Sauce

The name "Hush Puppies" is said to come from Southern cooks tossing bits of this fried dough to the noisy dogs and saying, "Hush, puppies!"

Yield: 28 Hush Puppies

- **½ cup Chipotle Dipping Sauce** **(pg. 292)**
- **½ cup finely minced onion**
- **1½ tsp. vegetable oil**
- **½ cup soy milk**
- **½ cup water**
- **¾ cup cornmeal**
- **½ cup plus 2 Tbs. flour**
- **¼ cup sugar**
- **1¼ tsp. salt**
- **1 tsp. baking powder**
- **½ tsp. garlic powder**
- **½ tsp. black pepper**
- **⅛ tsp. cayenne**
- **Vegetable oil, for frying**

Prepare Chipotle Dipping Sauce and set aside.

In a 3-quart saucepan, sauté the onion with the 1½ tsp. oil until tender.

Add soy milk and water and bring to a boil.

Whisk in cornmeal and cook until thickened (about one minute). Remove from heat, cover, and let sit for 20 minutes.

Transfer to a mixing bowl. Add remaining ingredients, except oil for frying, and mix until mixture comes together (mixture may seem dry at first).

Form into walnut-sized balls.

Preheat two inches of oil in a small saucepan or recommended amount of oil in a deep fat fryer to 350°F.

Fry hush puppies until golden brown and done in the middle, about three minutes.

Serve with dipping sauce on the side.

Jalapeño Pierogi

Pierogies, with their potato, cabbage, onion, and cheese filling, are mainly associated with Poland but variations are found around the world.

Yield: 18 boiled* or fried Pierogies**

1 batch Basic Dough (pg. 324)

4 cups peeled and diced potatoes

1 onion, small dice

1 fresh jalapeño, minced

1 Tbs. vegetable oil

1 cup vegan sour cream, divided

1 tsp. salt

¼ tsp. black pepper

Vegetable oil for baking or frying

Prepare Basic Dough. Cover and set aside.

Boil diced potatoes until soft. Drain off water, mash, and set aside.

Sauté the onion and jalapeño with the one Tbs. oil until tender. Stir in mashed potatoes, ¼ cup of the sour cream, salt, and black pepper.

Divide dough into 18 pieces.

Roll a single piece of dough into a 3-inch circle.

Place two Tbs. of filling on center of dough round.

Fold the dough over, forming a semi-circle. Press the edges together with the tines of a fork.

Repeat with remaining dough and filling.

Choose either the boiled or fried method below.

Serve cooked Pierogies with remaining sour cream on the side.

** Boiled method: In batches, place Pierogies in boiling water until the dough is cooked, about two or three minutes.*

*** Fried method:*
Preheat ¼-inch of oil in a skillet or recommended amount of oil in a deep fat fryer to 350°F.
Fry Pierogies until golden brown on each side, turning as necessary.

Pita Chips with Hummus

Yield: 3 servings

¾ cup Hummus (pg. 301)

3 Pitas (pg. 237)

¼ cup olive oil

1 tsp. curry powder

½ tsp. onion powder

¼ tsp. black pepper

¼ tsp. salt

Prepare Hummus and set aside.

Preheat oven to 425°F.

Brush pitas with olive oil.

In a small bowl, combine remaining ingredients.

Sprinkle seasoning over pita and re-brush to combine the seasoning with the oil.

Cut each pita into eight triangles.

Place triangles in a single layer on a baking sheet, cooking in batches if needed.

Bake for 10 minutes.

Serve with hummus.

Pot Stickers

Yield: 16

1 cup Asian Dipping Sauce (pg. 286) or favorite dipping sauce

16 Wonton Wrappers (pg. 340) or store bought vegan wonton wrappers

¾ cup shredded napa or green cabbage

¾ cup shredded carrot

2 Tbs. minced fresh ginger

1 Tbs. vegetable oil

4 oz. five spice baked tofu, shredded

1 bunch green onions, diced

Vegetable oil for grilling

Prepare Asian Dipping Sauce and set aside.

Prepare Wonton Wrappers and set aside.

In a frying pan, lightly sauté the cabbage, carrot, and ginger with one Tbs. oil. Transfer to a mixing bowl.

Add tofu and green onions.

Place two Tbs. of filling in the center of each wonton wrapper.

Fold the dough over, forming a semi-circle. Seal edges with a light amount of water.

Fill a large pot half full with water and bring to a boil.

Gently boil pot stickers (in batches, if needed, to prevent overcrowding) for five minutes.

Remove pot stickers from water and place on a plate.

In a large skillet or frying pan, grill one side of each pot sticker with oil until lightly browned.

Samosas with Potatoes and Peas

Samosas are a popular street food. Serve with Pita (pg. 237), Naan (pg. 236), Brown Rice (pg. 85), and/or Raita (pg. 312) if preferred.

Yield: 16 baked* or fried Samosas**

1 batch Basic Dough (pg. 324)

4 cups small diced peeled potatoes

1 small red onion, small dice

¼ cup olive oil

1½ cups fresh or frozen peas

2 Tbs. minced fresh ginger

1¼ tsp. garam masala

1 tsp. cumin powder

⅛ tsp. cayenne (optional)

Salt to taste (about 1¾ tsp.)

Vegetable oil for frying or baking

Prepare Basic Dough. Cover and set aside.

Boil potatoes just until tender. Drain off water and set potatoes aside until needed.

In a large pan, sauté the onion with the oil until tender. Add peas and ginger. Sauté one minute. Reduce heat to low.

On reduced heat, add garam masala, cumin, and cayenne. Sauté one minute. Add potatoes and sauté until warm.

Add salt to taste.

Place potato filling in refrigerator until chilled to room temperature.

Divide dough into 16 pieces.

On a lightly floured surface, roll a single piece of dough into a 4-inch circle.

Place three Tbs. of filling in middle of dough round.

Fold the dough over to form a semi-circle. Press the edges together with the tines of a fork.

Repeat with remaining dough and filling.

Choose either the baked or fried method below.

Samosas with Potatoes and Peas
(*continued*)

* *Baked method:*
Preheat oven to 425°F. Place Samosas in an oiled baking dish. Brush with oil and bake for 20 minutes.

** *Fried method:*
Preheat ¼-inch of oil in a skillet or recommended amount of oil in a deep fat fryer to 350°F. Fry Samosas until golden brown on each side, turning as necessary.

Japan

Sautéed Gingered Edamame

When serving and eating edamame, serve the whole pods but only eat the soybean inside the pod.

Yield: 3 servings

½ lb. frozen edamame in pod

1 Tbs. minced fresh ginger

2 Tbs. vegetable oil

2 Tbs. soy sauce

1 Tbs. sesame seeds

Bring four cups of water to a boil.

Place edamame in boiling water. Return water to a boil and boil for four minutes. Drain off water.

In a large frying pan, sauté the ginger with the oil until tender (about two minutes).

Add edamame, soy sauce, and sesame seeds and sauté one minute.

Spicy Black Bean Fritter with Chipotle Dipping Sauce

Yield: 24 fritters

1 cup Chipotle Dipping Sauce (pg. 292)

2 15-oz. cans black beans, drained and rinsed

2 Tbs. Chipotle Tabasco Sauce

2 Tbs. lime juice (about 1 lime)

2 Tbs. vegetable oil

2 tsp. salt

½ cup chopped onion

½ tsp. baking powder

¾ cup flour

Vegetable oil for frying

Prepare Chipotle Dipping Sauce and set aside.

In a food processor, process the black beans, Chipotle Tabasco Sauce, lime juice, two Tbs. oil, and salt until smooth.

Transfer mixture to a bowl. Stir in the onion, baking powder, and flour.

Pour the frying oil into a heavy-bottom pan until the oil is 1-inch deep.

Heat the oil to 350°F, checking the temperature with a candy thermometer. Watch oil temperature while cooking and adjust as necessary.

Carefully lower walnut-sized scoops of the bean mixture into the hot oil.

Fry fritters until browned and no longer doughy in the middle, about three to four minutes.

Drain on a plate lined with paper towels.

Serve with Chipotle Dipping Sauce on the side.

Spring Rolls

Serve with your favorite dipping sauce or Asian Dipping Sauce (pg. 286).

Yield: 12 rolls

12 rice paper wrappers*

6 oz. ready-to-serve teriyaki tofu, thin julienne cut

1 cup shredded napa cabbage

1 cup shredded carrot

½ bunch green onions, finely sliced

Dip one spring roll wrapper in very hot water (not boiling) until soft, about 10 seconds. Place on a slightly damp tea or dish towel.

Place ½ of each filling ingredient in the center of the wrapper and roll up burrito style. Repeat with remaining ingredients.

Serve cold with dipping sauce on the side.

* *Rice paper wrappers are also called rice paper, spring roll wrappers, or banh trang wrappers. They are paper-thin, translucent, usually round, and turn clear when soaked in hot water.*

Steamed Buns

Serve with Asian Dipping Sauce (pg. 286) or your favorite dipping sauce.

Yield: 16 buns

Dough:

1 Tbs. active dry yeast (1¼-oz. package)

1 tsp. sugar

1 cup warm water (110°F)

2¾ cup flour*

3 Tbs. vegetable oil

1¼ tsp. salt

Filling:

1 small onion, minced

2 small carrots, minced

1 cup minced celery

1½ cups minced green cabbage

¼ cup minced fresh ginger

2 Tbs. vegetable oil

1 Tbs. sesame oil

8 oz. ready-to-serve teriyaki tofu, small dice

¼ cup soy sauce

16 2-inch X 2-inch pieces of foil

** Use part whole wheat flour if you prefer.*

Dough:

In a large bowl, whisk together the yeast, sugar, and warm water and let sit for five minutes.

Add flour, the three Tbs. of vegetable oil, and salt.

On a floured surface, knead dough for seven minutes.

Place kneaded dough in a large, oiled bowl. Cover with clear wrap and let sit in a warm place until doubled in size.

While the dough is rising, make the filling.

Filling:

In a large pan, sauté the onion, carrots, celery, cabbage, and ginger with the two Tbs. vegetable oil and the sesame oil until tender.

Add tofu and soy sauce. Remove filling from pan and place in a shallow container to cool in refrigerator.

Assembling Steamed Buns:

Punch down dough and knead for one minute. Divide dough into 16 pieces.

Roll each piece of dough into a ball.

On a lightly floured surface, roll a single piece of dough into a 6-inch round.

Place ¼ cup of mixture in the middle of each dough round. Gather up the edges and twist to seal.

Place each bun, twisted side down, on a piece of foil.

Place a steam basket in a saucepan. Fill saucepan with water to just below the bottom of the steam basket. Bring water to a boil. Place buns with foil in steamer leaving a 1-inch space between buns. You may need to cook in batches if your steamer will not accommodate all of the buns at once. Cover with a tight-fitting lid and steam for 15 minutes.

Remove buns from steamer basket, remove foil, and serve with dipping sauce.

Tempura Onion Rings

Yield: 30 Rings

1 large sweet onion

1¼ cups flour

¼ cup cornstarch

1 Tbs. salt

2 tsp. baking powder

1¼ cups soy milk

Vegetable oil for frying

Peel onion. Slice into ½-inch thick whole rings. Separate rings and set aside the 30 largest rings for use.

In a large shallow bowl, whisk together the flour, cornstarch, salt, and baking powder.

Whisk in the soy milk.

Heat oil in deep fat fryer, or 1-inch of oil in a large, heavy bottom skillet to 350°F. Use a candy thermometer to check the temperature of the oil. Regulate heat while cooking to maintain a temperature range of 330°F - 370°F.

Lightly batter each onion ring and fry in oil until browned on each side, flipping once.

Place cooked onion rings on a plate lined with paper towels.

Repeat until all onion rings are cooked.

Thai Lettuce Wrap

Use only the best outer leaves for the wraps and do not overfill, or else they will be messy when eaten.

Yield: 12 wraps

¼ lb. Roasted Edamame (pg. 336)

½ cup Peanut Sauce (pg. 307)

12 large Bibb lettuce leaves

4 oz. ready-to-serve teriyaki tofu, thin julienne cut

½ cup shredded purple cabbage

½ cup shredded carrot

¼ cup finely chopped green onions

½ bunch basil, stemmed and julienne cut

¼ cup vegan sriracha sauce (optional)

Prepare roasted edamame and place in refrigerator to chill until needed.

Prepare Peanut Sauce and set aside.

Fill each lettuce leaf with tofu, roasted edamame, cabbage, carrot, green onion, basil, and drizzle with peanut sauce. Leave open-faced.

Serve vegan sriracha sauce on the side.

Thai Plantain Fritter

Serve with Peanut Sauce (pg. 307) if desired.

Yield: 8 fritters

2 green plantains

1 cup minced onion

3 Tbs. peanut butter

2 tsp. vegan sriracha sauce

¾ tsp. salt

Vegetable oil for grilling

Peel and shred plantains. Place in a mixing bowl.

Stir in minced onion, peanut butter, vegan sriracha sauce, and salt.

Form into eight ¾-inch thick round fritters.

Heat ¼-inch of oil in a frying pan. Grill fritters until crisp and browned on each side.

Serve with additional vegan sriracha sauce if preferred.

Soups:

African Peanut Soup

Traditionally served with Fufu Soup Bowl (pg. 91)

Yield: 6 servings

1 small onion, small dice

1¼ cups small diced yam

3 Tbs. vegetable oil

2 Tbs. flour

1 cup vegetable broth

14-oz. can unsweetened coconut milk

1½ cups diced tomatoes or 1 15-oz. can diced tomatoes

½ cup crunchy unsweetened peanut butter

¼ tsp. ground black pepper

Salt to taste (about 1½ tsp.)

In a 3-quart saucepan, sauté the onion and yam with the oil until tender.

Stir in flour.

Add vegetable broth, coconut milk, and diced tomatoes. Simmer for 10 minutes.

Stir in peanut butter and black pepper.

Add salt to taste.

Serve in Fufu Soup Bowl if desired.

Borscht

Yield: 4 servings

4 cups vegetable broth

3 small red potatoes, medium dice

1 cup peeled and shredded fresh beets

1 carrot, medium dice

1 cup shredded green cabbage

¼ cup chopped fresh dill or 2 tsp. dry

Salt to taste (about ½ tsp.)

½ cup vegan sour cream for serving

In a 3-quart covered saucepan, boil potatoes, beets, carrot, and cabbage in vegetable broth just until tender, about 15 minutes.

Add dill and cook one minute.

Add salt to taste.

Serve soup in individual serving bowls and add two Tbs. sour cream to each bowl.

Canadian Barley Soup

Canada is a leading producer of barley.

Yield: 4 servings

⅓ cup uncooked barley, rinsed

4 cups vegetable broth

3 carrots, small dice

4 stalks celery, small dice

½ onion, small dice

3 Tbs. vegetable oil

2 medium tomatoes, small dice

3 Tbs. flour

1 tsp. onion powder

⅛ tsp. black pepper

Salt to taste (about 2 tsp.)

In a 3-quart saucepan, add barley and vegetable broth. Bring to a boil, reduce heat to low, cover and simmer until barley is soft, about 45 minutes. Set aside.

In a large pot, sauté the carrots, celery, and onion with the oil until tender. Add tomatoes and cook for one minute. Reduce heat to low.

On reduced heat, add the flour, onion powder, and black pepper and sauté for one minute.

Add the cooked barley and vegetable broth.

Heat soup on medium-high heat until hot and thickened, stirring frequently.

Add salt to taste.

Chili Sin Carne

Chili Sin Carne translates to "Chili without Meat."

Yield: 4 servings

½ onion, small dice

2 Tbs. vegetable oil

1½ tsp. chili powder

1½ tsp. onion powder

½ tsp. sugar

15-oz. can pinto beans, drained and rinsed

15-oz. can tomato sauce

¼ cup water

2 Tbs. TVP (textured vegetable protein) (optional)

Salt to taste (about ¾ tsp.)

In a 2-quart saucepan, sauté the onion with the oil until tender. Reduce heat to low.

Add chili powder, onion powder, and sugar and sauté for one minute.

Add beans, tomato sauce, water, and TVP.

Simmer on medium-low heat for 10 minutes, stirring occasionally.

Add salt to taste.

Creamy Tomato Soup

Yield: 4 servings

2 6-oz. cans tomato paste

1¼ cups unsweetened soy milk

2 cups vegetable broth

1½ tsp. sugar

Salt to taste (about 1 tsp.)

Pepper to taste (about ¼ tsp.)

In a 3-quart saucepan, whisk together tomato paste, soy milk, vegetable broth, and sugar.

Heat until hot, stirring frequently.

Add salt and pepper to taste.

Hominy and Barley Soup

Use either white or golden hominy.

Yield: 6 servings

¼ cup uncooked barley, rinsed

4 cups vegetable broth

3 carrots, small dice

4 stalks celery, small dice

½ onion, small dice

3 Tbs. vegetable oil

2 Tbs. flour

1 tsp. onion powder

½ tsp. chili powder

½ tsp. cumin

¼ tsp. thyme

⅛ tsp. black pepper

2 15-oz. cans hominy, drained and rinsed

3 Tbs. tomato paste

Salt to taste (about 1½ tsp.)

In a 3-quart saucepan, add barley and vegetable broth. Bring to a boil, reduce heat to low, cover, and simmer until barley is soft, about 45 minutes. Set aside.

In a large pot, sauté the carrots, celery, and onion with the oil until tender. Reduce heat to low.

Add the flour, onion powder, chili powder, cumin, thyme, and black pepper and sauté for one minute.

Add the cooked barley, vegetable broth, hominy, and tomato paste.

Heat soup on medium-high heat until hot, stirring often.

Add salt to taste.

Southern USA

Hoppin' John Soup

Black-eyed peas are a traditional good luck ingredient in New Year's Day meals.

Yield: 6 servings

1 small onion, small dice

1 small red bell pepper, small dice

4 stalks celery, small dice

3 Tbs. vegetable oil

14 oz. vegan breakfast-style sausage

1 cup dry black-eyed peas

4 cups vegetable broth

1 tomato, small dice

2 Tbs. uncooked brown rice

Salt to taste (about ½ tsp.)

Pepper to taste (about ¼ tsp.)

In a large stockpot, sauté the onion, bell pepper, and celery with the oil until tender.

Add sausage and continue to cook until sausage is broken-up and browned.

Add black-eyed peas, vegetable broth, tomato, and rice.

Bring soup to a boil.

Reduce heat to low. Cover and simmer for one hour or until beans and rice are tender, stirring occasionally.

Add salt and pepper to taste.

Hot and Sour Soup

Yield: 5 servings

1 carrot cut into thin julienne strips

½ pound sliced mushrooms

2 cups shredded green cabbage

1 bunch green onions, chopped

2 Tbs. sesame oil

4 cups mushroom or vegetable broth

8-oz. can bamboo shoots, drained and cut into thin julienne strips

½ cup soy sauce

3 Tbs. sugar

2 Tbs. rice vinegar

¼ tsp. black pepper

3 Tbs. cornstarch

¼ cup cold water

16 oz. firm tofu, cut into julienne strips

Cayenne pepper to taste (about ¼ tsp.)

Salt to taste (about 1 tsp.)

In a large stock pot, sauté the carrot, mushrooms, cabbage, and green onions with the sesame oil until tender.

Add broth, bamboo shoots, soy sauce, sugar, rice vinegar, and black pepper.

Bring soup to a boil.

In a small bowl, combine cornstarch and water. While stirring soup, slowly add cornstarch mixture.

Add tofu. Heat soup until hot and thickened.

Add cayenne pepper and salt to taste.

Hungarian Goulash

This recipe is the Paprikás Krumpli (paprika and potatoes) version of goulash.

Yield: 4 servings

1 onion, medium dice

2 carrots, medium dice

3 stalks celery, medium dice

3 Tbs. vegetable oil

3 Tbs. Hungarian sweet paprika

3 Tbs. flour

2 medium potatoes, medium dice

1 tomato, medium dice

3 cups vegetable broth

Black pepper to taste (about ¼ tsp.)

Salt to taste (about 1½ tsp.)

In a large stockpot, sauté the onion, carrots, and celery with the oil until tender.

Add paprika and flour.

Add potatoes, tomato, and broth.

Bring to a boil, reduce heat to low, cover, and simmer until potatoes are tender (about 30 minutes).

Add salt and pepper to taste.

Irish Stew

The Irish call potatoes "spuds," a reference to the type of shovel used to dig potatoes.

Yield: 6 servings

4 small russet potatoes, peeled and large dice

4 carrots, large dice

4 stalks of celery, large dice

1 onion, large dice

½ cup vegetable oil

¾ cup flour

1 tsp. onion powder

¼ tsp. thyme

15-oz. can white beans, drained and rinsed

4 cups vegetable broth

Salt to taste (about 2 tsp.)

Pepper to taste (about ¼ tsp.)

Boil potatoes just until soft but not mushy. Drain off water and set potatoes aside.

In a large saucepan, sauté the carrots, celery, and onion with the oil until tender. Reduce heat to low.

Add flour, onion powder and thyme. Sauté for one minute.

Increase heat to medium. Add beans, vegetable broth, and cooked potatoes. Heat until hot and thickened, stirring frequently.

Add salt and pepper to taste.

Italian Wedding Soup

Yield: 6 servings

12 Meatballs (pg. 329)

2 carrots, small dice

3 stalks celery, small dice

½ onion, small dice

3 Tbs. vegetable oil

1 tsp. basil

1 tsp. oregano

1 tsp. garlic powder

1 tsp. onion powder

4 cups vegetable broth

½ cup uncooked elbow macaroni

1 bunch escarole or ½ bunch spinach, chopped

Salt to taste (about 1½ tsp.)

Prepare Meatballs. Quarter meatballs and set aside.

In a large pot, sauté the carrots, celery and onion with the oil until tender.

Add basil, oregano, garlic powder and onion powder. Cook for one minute.

Add vegetable broth and escarole or spinach.

Bring to a boil. Stir in pasta. Cook until pasta is soft, stirring often.

Add meatballs and cook until hot.

Add salt to taste.

Jamaican Coconut and Bean Soup

Yield: 5 servings

2 carrots, small dice

4 stalks celery, small dice

1 small onion, small dice

¼ cup vegetable oil

½ tsp. thyme

½ tsp. garlic powder

½ tsp. onion powder

⅓ cup flour

1 cup vegetable broth

2 15-oz. cans unsweetened coconut milk

16-oz. can kidney beans, drained and rinsed

Zest of 2 limes

Juice of 2 limes

Salt to taste (about 1½ tsp.)

Black pepper to taste (about ¼ tsp.)

In a 3-quart saucepan, sauté the carrots, celery, and onion with the oil until tender. Reduce heat to low.

On reduced heat, add thyme, garlic powder, onion powder, and flour. Sauté for one minute, stirring constantly.

Add the vegetable broth, coconut milk, kidney beans, lime zest, and lime juice.

Heat soup on medium-high heat until hot and thickened, stirring often.

Add salt and pepper to taste.

Japan

Miso Soba Noodle Soup

Soba noodles, which contain buckwheat, provide high nutritional value.

Yield: 4 servings

3 oz. soba noodles (uncooked)

4 cups water

½ cup miso paste

8 oz. extra firm tofu, medium dice

Soy sauce to taste (about 2 Tbs.)

Topping options:
bean sprouts, chopped cilantro, chopped jalapeños, lime wedges, green onions, red pepper flakes, shredded carrot, julienned red pepper

Cook soba noodles according to package directions and set aside.

In a 3-quart saucepan, combine water and miso paste. Bring to a boil.

Add tofu and simmer for five minutes.

Add cooked soba noodles.

Add soy sauce to taste.

Add toppings.

Mulligatawny Soup

"Mulligatawny" means pepper water in Tamil.

Yield: 4 servings

2 cups water

¼ cup uncooked green lentils, rinsed

¼ cup uncooked brown rice

1 carrot, medium dice

2 stalks celery, medium dice

½ onion, small dice

1 green apple, peeled, cored, and small dice

1 jalapeño pepper, mince

3 Tbs. vegetable oil

2 Tbs. curry powder

2 Tbs. flour

14-oz. can unsweetened coconut milk

15-oz. can diced tomatoes

Salt to taste

1 bunch cilantro, chopped

In a 2-quart saucepan combine water, lentils, and rice. Bring to a boil and reduce heat to low. Cover and simmer until lentils and rice are soft, about 50 minutes. Set aside (do not drain).

In a 3-quart saucepan, sauté the carrot, celery, onion, apple, and jalapeño with the oil until tender.

Add curry powder and flour.

Add coconut milk, diced tomatoes, and cooked lentils/rice/water.

Bring to a boil. Reduce heat and simmer for 10 minutes.

Add salt to taste.

Top with cilantro.

Vietnam

Pho Noodle Bowl

Pho, pronounced "fuh," is a clear broth soup made with simple ingredients and finished with a variety of fresh and flavorful toppings.

Yield: 3 servings

1 sachet bag or cheesecloth

4 whole star anise

2-inch cinnamon stick

10 whole cloves

1 small red onion, small dice

½ lb. crimini mushrooms, sliced

2 Tbs. minced ginger

1 tsp. vegetable oil

4 cups vegetable broth

¼ cup soy sauce

1 cup shelled edamame

3 oz. uncooked soba noodles

Salt to taste (if needed)

Topping options:
green onions, basil, bean sprouts, shredded cabbage, mint, cilantro, jalapeños, lime wedges

Wrap star anise, cinnamon stick, and cloves in a sachet bag or cheesecloth and tie off. Set aside.

In a large pot, sauté the onion, mushrooms, and ginger with the oil until tender.

Add vegetable broth, soy sauce, edamame, and sachet.

Bring to a boil, cover, and simmer for 20 minutes.

Remove sachet bag.

Bring soup to a boil.

Add soba noodles. Cook until noodles are tender, stirring often.

Add salt to taste if needed.

Add toppings of choice.

Russian Potato Mushroom Soup

Yield: 4 servings

- 4 small red potatoes, medium dice
- ½ cup potato water (see instructions)
- 2 cups chopped leeks
- 4 cups sliced mushrooms (about 1 lb.)
- ¼ cup vegetable oil
- 1 tsp. dill
- ¼ cup flour
- 1½ cups plain unsweetened soy milk
- 12 oz. vegan sour cream
- Salt to taste (about 1 tsp.)
- Pepper to taste (about ¼ tsp.)

Boil potatoes just until tender. Save ½ cup of the potato cooking water. Drain off remaining water. Set potatoes and the ½ cup of potato water aside.

In a 3-quart saucepan, sauté the leeks and mushrooms with the oil until tender.

Add dill and flour and cook for one minute.

Add soy milk, sour cream, and the ½ cup of potato water. Cook until hot and thickened, stirring constantly.

Add cooked potatoes and heat until hot.

Add salt and pepper to taste.

Scotch Broth

Yield: 6 servings

4 stalks celery, medium dice

3 carrots, medium dice

1 onion, medium dice

1 turnip, medium dice

½ cup uncooked barley, rinsed

14-oz. can diced tomatoes

15-oz. can kidney beans, drained and rinsed

4 cups vegetable broth

Salt to taste (about 2 tsp.)

Pepper to taste (about ¼ tsp.)

In a large pot, add all ingredients except salt and pepper.

Bring to a boil, reduce heat to low, cover and simmer until barley is cooked, about 45 minutes.

Add salt and pepper to taste.

Spicy Carrot Ginger Coconut Soup

Yield: 5 servings

3 cups small diced carrots

½ sweet onion, small dice

¼ cup olive oil

¼ cup minced ginger

¼ cup flour

12-oz. can unsweetened coconut milk

¼ cup frozen orange juice concentrate

2 cups vegetable broth

2 Tbs. soy sauce

⅛ tsp. cayenne pepper (optional)

Salt to taste (about 1½ tsp.)

In a large stockpot, sauté the carrots and onion with the oil until tender. Add ginger and continue to sauté until ginger is tender. Reduce heat to low.

Add flour and sauté for one minute.

Add coconut milk, orange juice concentrate, vegetable broth, soy sauce, and cayenne pepper.

Bring to a boil. Reduce heat to low. Cover and simmer for 15 minutes, stirring occasionally.

Carefully puree soup in a blender.

Reheat if needed.

Add salt to taste.

Thai Coconut Squash Soup

Yield: 5 servings

1 small butternut squash, peeled, seeded, and medium dice

1 medium sweet onion, small dice

¼ cup vegetable oil

¼ cup fresh peeled and minced ginger

2 cups vegetable broth

14-oz. can unsweetened coconut milk

Salt to taste (about 1½ tsp.)

Boil butternut squash until tender. Discard water and set squash aside.

In a 3-quart saucepan, sauté the onion with the oil until tender. Reduce heat to low.

Add ginger and cook until ginger is tender, about five minutes.

Add flour and cook one minute.

Add vegetable broth, coconut milk, and squash.

On medium-high heat, bring soup to a boil, stirring constantly.

Add salt to taste.

Turkish Bean Soup

Yield: 5 servings

2 carrots, small dice

3 stalks celery, small dice

½ onion, small dice

¼ cup vegetable oil

½ tsp. thyme

½ tsp. onion powder

¼ tsp. black pepper

¼ tsp. red pepper flakes

¼ cup flour

4 cups vegetable broth

2 15-oz. cans white beans, drained and rinsed

⅓ cup tomato paste

Salt to taste (about 1½ tsp.)

In a large pot, sauté the carrots, celery, and onion with the oil until tender. Reduce heat to low.

Add thyme, onion powder, black pepper, red pepper flakes, and flour and sauté one minute.

Add vegetable broth, beans, and tomato paste.

Heat soup on medium-high heat until hot and thickened, stirring often.

Add salt to taste.

Salads:

Barley Salad

Yield: 8 servings

1 cup uncooked barley, rinsed

¼ cup olive oil

1 bunch fresh basil, stems removed and leaves chopped

2 medium tomatoes, medium dice

½ bunch green onions, small dice

¼ cup lemon juice

Salt to taste (about ¾ tsp.)

Black pepper to taste (about ¼ tsp.)

Boil barley until tender, about 45 minutes. Drain off water and rinse with cold water until cool. Drain well and toss with olive oil.

Add basil, tomatoes, green onions, and lemon juice.

Add salt and pepper to taste.

Chill before serving.

Black Bean and Corn Salad

Black beans were domesticated in ancient Central America.

Yield: 8 servings

3 ears of corn

15-oz. can black beans, drained and rinsed

1 tomato, medium dice

1 bunch cilantro, chopped

1 red bell pepper, small dice

¼ cup vegan Mayonnaise (pg. 304)

Juice of 1 lime

Salt to taste (about 1½ tsp.)

Boil corn for 10 minutes. Remove the corn from the boiling water. Run cold water over the corn to stop the cooking process and to chill the corn.

Cut the kernels off the cob and place kernels in a large bowl.

Add remaining ingredients, except salt, and toss.

Add salt to taste.

Chill before serving.

Caesar Pasta Salad

Caesar Salad is generally attributed to Italian-born restaurateur Caesar Cardini. Ironically, Cardini opposed the use of anchovies in his salad, which has kept it out of reach of vegetarians for years.

Yield: 6 servings

8 oz. uncooked penne pasta

1 cup Caesar Salad Dressing (pg. 78)

8 whole olives, sliced

14 oz. can quartered artichoke hearts, drained

½ small red onion, thinly sliced

6 cups chopped romaine

3 cups Croutons (pg. 326)

Cook pasta according to package instructions. Drain off pasta water. Rinse pasta with cold water until cool, drain thoroughly, and place in a large bowl.

Stir in Caesar salad dressing, sliced olives, artichoke hearts, and red onion.

Serve pasta mixture on a bed of chopped romaine.

Top with croutons.

Cannellini Bean Salad

Yield: 8 servings

2 15-oz. cans cannellini beans, drained and rinsed

14-oz. can quartered artichoke hearts, drained and lightly chopped

4-oz. can sliced black olives, drained

½ red onion, thinly sliced

½ cup chopped fresh parsley

½ cup balsamic vinegar

¼ cup olive oil

Salt to taste (about 1½ tsp.)

Pepper to taste (about ¼ tsp.)

In a large bowl, combine all ingredients except salt and pepper.

Add salt and pepper to taste.

Let marinate for a minimum of 30 minutes.

Cilantro Lime Slaw

Yield: 6 servings

In a large bowl, combine all ingredients.

6 cups shredded cabbage

1 red bell pepper, thinly sliced

½ red onion, thinly sliced

2 bunches cilantro, chopped

1 cup vegan Mayonnaise (pg. 304)

Juice of 2 limes

¼ cup sugar

½ tsp. salt

Cucumber Salad

Yield: 6 servings

2 cucumbers, peeled, seeded, and medium dice

1 tomato, medium dice

½ cup chopped red onion

½ bunch parsley, chopped

½ cup rice vinegar

2 Tbs. red wine vinegar

3 Tbs. olive oil

2 tsp. salt

⅛ tsp. black pepper

In a large bowl, combine all ingredients.

Marinate in refrigerator for one hour.

Drain off marinade before serving.

Falafel Salad

Yield: 6 servings

2 cups Tzatziki Sauce (pg. 321)

Pita Chips (pg. 18)

1 batch Falafel (pg. 160)

1 head romaine or iceberg lettuce, shredded

2 tomatoes, medium dice

24 Kalamata olives, pitted and halved

14-oz. jar artichoke hearts, drained and quartered

½ red onion cut into thinly sliced rings

1 cucumber, peeled, seeded, and medium dice

½ cup roasted salted sunflower seeds

Prepare Tzatziki Sauce and set aside.

Prepare Pita Chips and set aside.

Prepare Falafel according to directions.

On a bed of greens arrange the Falafel, tomatoes, olives, artichokes, onions, and cucumber.

Top with sunflower seeds, Tzatziki Sauce, and Pita Chips.

French Green Lentil and Bulgur Salad

Bulgur is often confused with cracked wheat, which is not par-cooked.

Yield: 4 servings

½ cup uncooked bulgur

¾ cup warm water

Juice of 2 limes

½ cup French green lentils, sorted and rinsed

1 bunch cilantro, stemmed and chopped

1 tomato, medium dice

3 Tbs. olive oil

Salt to taste (about 1 tsp.)

Soak bulgur in warm water and lime juice until tender, about one hour. Drain off liquid.

While bulgur is soaking, boil lentils until tender but not mushy, about 20 minutes. Drain and chill.

In a bowl, combine bulgur, lentils, cilantro, tomato, and oil.

Add salt to taste.

German Potato Salad

Yield: 4 servings

4 large red potatoes, large dice

½ onion, small dice

2 Tbs. vegetable oil

2 Tbs. apple cider vinegar

1 Tbs. brown sugar

Salt to taste (about ¾ tsp.)

Pepper to taste (about ½ tsp.)

Boil potatoes just until tender. Drain and chill potatoes.

In a large skillet, sauté the onion with the oil until tender. Add potatoes and sauté until browned, being careful not to mash up potatoes.

Add apple cider vinegar and brown sugar.

Add salt and pepper to taste.

Serve warm or cold.

Hawaiian Potato Macaroni Salad

Yield: 6 servings

4 medium russet potatoes, whole and unpeeled

1¼ cups uncooked macaroni

3 stalks celery, small dice

½ sweet onion, small dice

1 cup vegan Mayonnaise (pg. 304)

1 cup chopped dill pickles

2 Tbs. prepared yellow mustard

Salt to taste (about 2 tsp.)

Pepper to taste (about ¼ tsp.)

Boil whole potatoes just until tender. Drain and cool for 15 minutes.

Peel potatoes while still warm.

Medium dice potatoes and then place in the refrigerator to chill.

Cook pasta according to package directions. Drain pasta and rinse with cold water. Place pasta in a large mixing bowl.

Add chilled diced potatoes, celery, onion, mayonnaise, chopped pickles, and mustard.

Add salt and pepper to taste.

Incan Quinoa Salad

Quinoa, which can be grown in the high altitudes of the Andes, is seen as a sacred crop. Quinoa contains essential amino acids, calcium, protein, fiber, and carbohydrates.

Yield: 10 servings

1 cup uncooked quinoa, rinsed

1½ cups water

1 cup pumpkin seeds (raw or toasted)

1 cup sliced almonds (raw or toasted)

1 cup dried fruit of choice (e.g. raisins, blueberries, cranberries, cherries, chopped apricots, chopped figs, date pieces)

2 Tbs. chopped fresh mint leaves

Zest of 2 limes, minced

Juice of 2 limes

2 Tbs. vegetable oil

1 Tbs. sugar

Salt to taste (about ½ tsp.)

In a 3-quart saucepan, bring quinoa and water to a boil. Reduce heat to low, cover, and simmer until quinoa is tender, about 18-20 minutes. Chill in refrigerator.

In large bowl, combine quinoa, pumpkin seeds, almonds, dried fruit, fresh mint, lime zest, lime juice, oil, and sugar.

Add salt to taste.

Lemon Wheat Berry Salad

Yield: 6 servings

2 cups uncooked wheat berries, rinsed

Juice of two lemons (½ cup)

3 Tbs. olive oil

½ cup chopped parsley

½ cup small diced red onion

Salt to taste (about 1 tsp.)

Place wheat berries in boiling water. Cover and simmer until tender, about one hour.

Drain off water and chill wheat berries.

In a bowl, combine wheat berries, lemon juice, olive oil, parsley, and red onion.

Add salt to taste.

England

Malt Vinegar Black Barley Salad

Yield: 6 servings

¾ cup uncooked black barley, rinsed

1 red bell pepper, small dice

15-oz. can lima beans, drained and rinsed

¼ cup malt vinegar

3 Tbs. olive oil

Salt to taste (about 1 tsp.)

Pepper to taste (about ¼ tsp.)

Boil barley until tender, about 45 minutes. Drain and rinse with cold water until chilled.

In a large bowl, combine barley, bell pepper, lima beans, malt vinegar, and olive oil.

Add salt and pepper to taste.

Mexican Salad

Yield: 6 servings

2 cups Avocado Dressing (pg. 76)

1 head iceberg lettuce, shredded

15-oz. can pinto beans, drained, rinsed, and chilled

15-oz. can golden hominy, drained, rinsed, and chilled

1 bunch green onions, chopped

1 red bell pepper, small dice

In a large bowl toss all ingredients except dressing.

Serve with dressing.

Italy

Panzanella Salad

Panzanella originated in the regions of Tuscany, Umbria, Marche, and Lazio. It is often made with untoasted bread.

Yield: 6 servings

White Balsamic Vinaigrette (pg. 81) or Italian Dressing to taste

16-oz. baguette, large dice

¼ cup olive oil

1 tsp. garlic powder

1 tsp. onion powder

1 tsp. salt

2 tomatoes, medium dice

1 bunch basil leaves, stemmed and lightly chopped

½ small red onion, thinly sliced

1 cucumber, peeled, seeded, medium dice

Optional ingredients:
olives, capers, roasted garlic, bell pepper, arugula, romaine hearts, baby spinach, fresh mint, fresh parsley, fresh tarragon

Preheat oven to 400°F.

In a large roasting pan, combine baguette pieces, olive oil, garlic powder, onion powder, and salt.

Bake for 10 minutes, stirring at five minutes, or leave unbaked if you prefer.

Cool to room temperature.

In a large bowl, combine baguette, tomatoes, basil, onion, cucumber, and any optional ingredients.

Toss with dressing just before serving.

Quinoa Tabbouleh Salad

Yield: 8 servings

1 cup uncooked quinoa, rinsed

1½ cups water

1 bunch fresh mint, stemmed and chopped

1 bunch fresh parsley, chopped

2 medium tomatoes, medium dice

½ bunch green onions, chopped

¼ cup lemon juice

⅓ cup olive oil

Salt to taste (about ¾ tsp.)

Black pepper to taste (about ¼ tsp.)

In a 3-quart saucepan, bring quinoa and water to a boil. Reduce heat to low, cover, and simmer until quinoa is tender, about 18-20 minutes. Chill in refrigerator.

Place chilled quinoa in a bowl. Add the mint, parsley, tomatoes, green onions, lemon juice, and olive oil.

Add salt and pepper to taste.

Sunomono

Yield: 6 servings

2 cucumbers, peeled, seeded, halved, and cut into ¼-inch slices

¾ cup seasoned rice vinegar

3 Tbs. sugar

2 tsp. salt

1 Tbs. minced fresh ginger

Combine all ingredients.

Marinate in refrigerator one hour before serving.

Thai Pineapple Salad

Yield: 4 servings

1 pineapple, peeled, cored, and medium dice

1 shredded carrot

1 cup shredded purple cabbage

¼ cup chopped fresh basil leaves

2 Tbs. vegan sriracha sauce

2 Tbs. sugar

Juice of one lime

Combine all ingredients.

Vegetable Quinoa Salad

Yield: 6 servings

1 cup uncooked quinoa, rinsed

1½ cups water

1 cup chopped broccoli

½ cup shredded carrot

¼ cup chopped onion

1 cup toasted slivered almonds

½ cup chopped pitted dates

¼ cup lemon juice

2 Tbs. olive oil

¼ tsp. ground black pepper

Salt to taste

In a small saucepan, combine quinoa and water. Bring to a boil, reduce heat to low, cover, and simmer until quinoa is tender, about 18-20 minutes.

Chill quinoa.

To the quinoa add remaining ingredients except salt.

Add salt to taste.

Yakisoba Noodle Salad

Yield: 6 servings

2 cups Black Sesame Seed Dressing (pg. 77)

12 oz. refrigerated precooked yakisoba noodles

1 bunch green onions, chopped

2 cups julienne cut snow peas

1 red bell pepper, small dice

Place yakisoba noodles in boiling water for one minute. Drain and rinse with cold water to chill noodles. Drain off water.

Chop noodles into bite-sized pieces.

In a large bowl, combine noodles, green onions, snow peas, and bell pepper.

Serve with dressing.

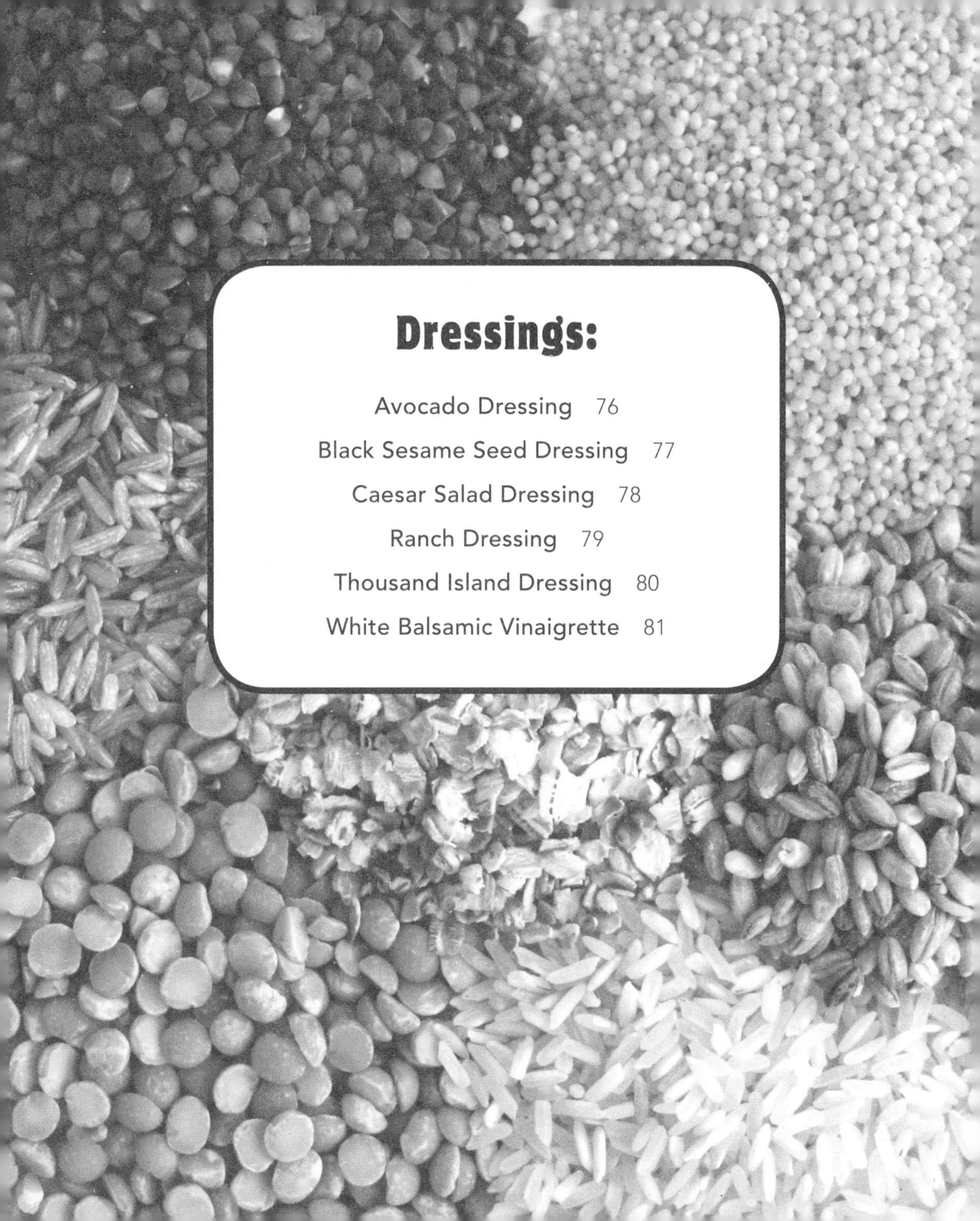

Dressings:

Avocado Dressing

Yield: 2 cups

2 ripe avocadoes, peeled and pitted

½ cup vegan sour cream

Juice of one lime

½ tsp. salt

Soy milk as needed

In a food processor, process all ingredients until smooth.

Add soy milk to thin dressing if preferred.

Black Sesame Seed Dressing

Yield: 1½ cups

¾ cup seasoned rice vinegar

½ cup vegan Mayonnaise (pg. 304)

¼ cup lemon juice

¼ cup sugar

2 Tbs. black sesame seeds

1 Tbs. soy sauce

1 Tbs. sesame oil

Whisk together all ingredients.

Caesar Salad Dressing

Yield: 1 cup

¾ cup vegan Mayonnaise (pg. 304)

Juice of 1 lemon (¼ cup)

2 tsp. vegan Worcestershire Sauce (pg. 322)

¾ tsp. black pepper

¼ tsp. salt

Whisk together all ingredients.

Ranch Dressing

Developed by Steve Henson in Alaska and later served to guests at his and wife's Hidden Valley Ranch in California.

Yield: 1¾ cups

.1 cup vegan Mayonnaise (pg. 304)

½ cup vegan sour cream

3 Tbs. apple cider vinegar

2 Tbs. soy milk

1¼ tsp. onion powder

¾ tsp. salt

¼ tsp. black pepper

Whisk together all ingredients.

USA

Thousand Island Dressing

Named for the Thousand Islands region of upstate New York.

Yield: 1 cup

½ cup vegan Mayonnaise (pg. 304)

¼ cup ketchup

¼ cup sweet relish

1 Tbs. lemon juice

Pinch of salt and pepper

Whisk together all ingredients.

White Balsamic Vinaigrette

Yield: 1¼ cups

¾ cup olive oil

½ cup white balsamic vinegar*

2 tsp. Dijon mustard

1 Tbs. sugar

1½ tsp. salt

¼ tsp. black pepper

Use a blender to emulsify (mixing oil and vinegar so they will not separate) all ingredients for one minute.

** Use different vinegar if preferred.*

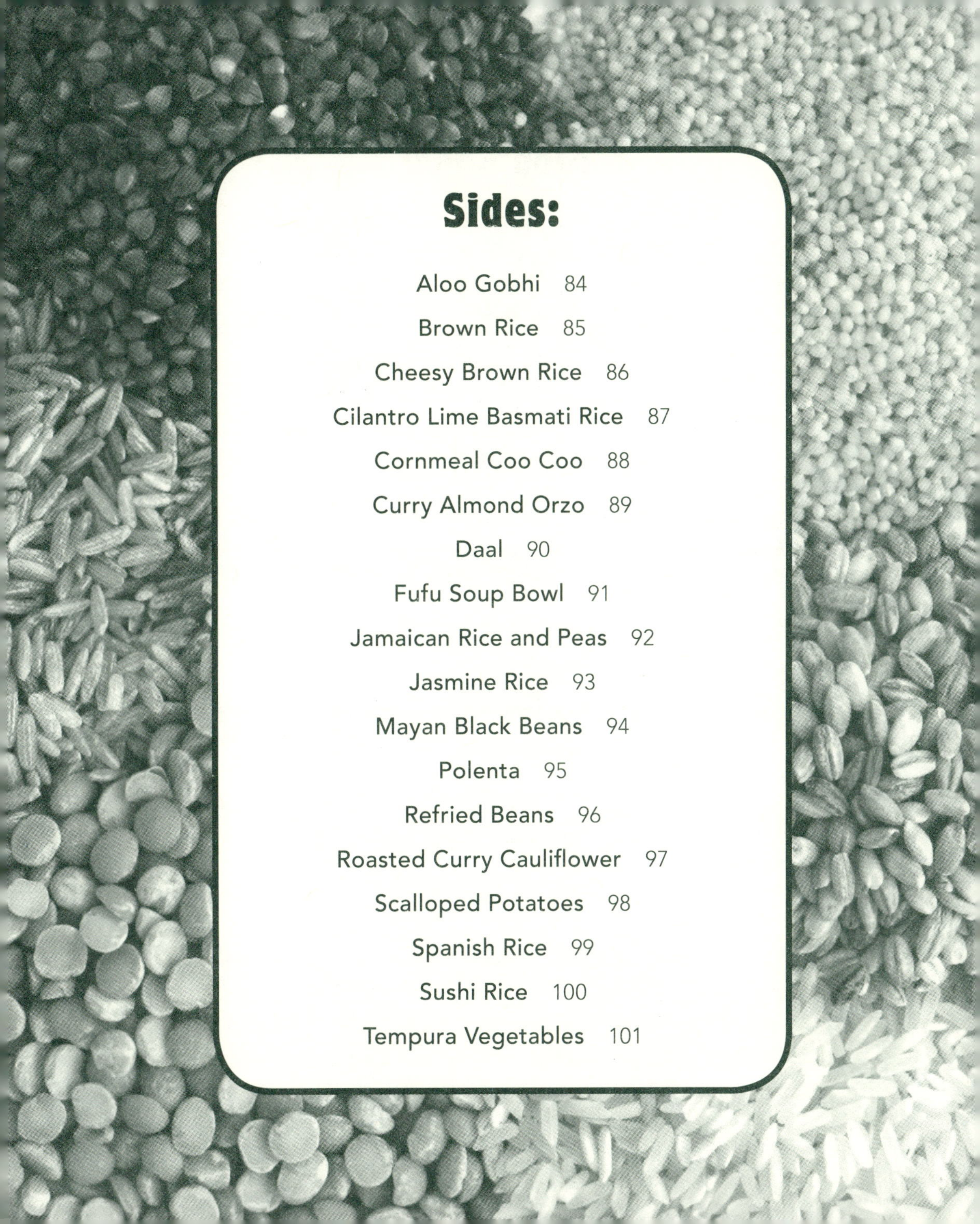

Sides:

Aloo Gobhi

Serve with Pita (pg. 237), Naan (pg. 236), or Brown Rice (pg. 85) if preferred.

Yield: 6 servings

4 cups peeled and medium diced russet potatoes

1 head of cauliflower cut into bite-sized pieces

½ red onion, small dice

⅓ cup olive oil

2 Tbs. minced fresh ginger

1 tsp. curry powder

½ tsp. garam masala

15-oz. can diced tomatoes

Salt to taste (about 2 tsp.)

1 bunch cilantro, chopped

Boil potatoes until soft but not mushy, about 15 minutes. Drain and set aside.

Boil cauliflower until soft but not mushy, about five minutes. Drain and set aside.

In a large pan, sauté the onion with the oil until tender.

Add ginger and cook until tender, about three minutes.

Add curry powder and garam masala. Cook for one minute.

Add tomatoes and cook for two minutes.

Add potatoes and cauliflower.

Simmer until hot, stirring frequently.

Add salt to taste.

Garnish with cilantro.

Brown Rice

Yield: 4 cups

1¼ cups long grain brown rice, rinsed and drained

2¼ cups water

In a 3-quart saucepan, bring rice and water to a boil.

Reduce heat to low, cover, and simmer until rice is tender, about 45 minutes.

Cheesy Brown Rice

Yield: 5 servings

4 cups cooked brown rice (pg. 85)

3 Tbs. vegetable oil

¼ cup flour

2 cups soy milk

½ cup nutritional yeast flakes

2 Tbs. nut butter of choice (for example, peanut, almond, etc.)

½ tsp. onion powder

½ tsp. paprika

Salt to taste (about 1¼ tsp.)

Prepare rice and set aside.

In a 3-quart saucepan, combine oil and flour. Heat on medium heat, stirring constantly, until bubbling.

Add remaining ingredients except salt and rice.

Heat sauce until hot and thickened, stirring constantly.

Combine cooked rice and cheese sauce.

Add salt to taste.

Cilantro Lime Basmati Rice

Yield: 4 cups

1¼ cups white basmati rice, rinsed

2½ cups water

½ cup chopped cilantro

Zest of one lime, minced

Juice of one lime

In a 2-quart saucepan, combine rice and water.

Bring to a boil, reduce heat to low, cover and simmer for 20 minutes or until rice is tender.

In a large bowl, combine cooked rice, cilantro, lime zest, and lime juice.

Cornmeal Coo Coo

Yield: 4 servings

2 cups water

8 frozen okras, thawed and dice small

3 Tbs. vegan margarine

½ tsp. salt

¼ tsp. black pepper

¾ cup cornmeal

In a 3-quart saucepan, add water, okra, margarine, salt, and pepper.

Bring to a boil.

Reduce heat to low and whisk in cornmeal.

Cook at low heat for five minutes, stirring frequently.

Remove from heat and cover with tight-fitting lid for 10 minutes.

Pour into oiled muffin cups.

Chill until set, about one hour.

Preheat oven to 325°F.

Bake for 15 minutes.

Curry Almond Orzo

Yield: 5 servings

8 oz. orzo

2 Tbs. olive oil

1 tsp. curry powder

Salt to taste (about ½ tsp.)

½ cup toasted sliced almonds

Boil orzo according to package instructions.

Strain and rinse with hot tap water.

Return to pan.

Stir in oil and curry powder.

Heat until hot.

Add salt to taste.

Top with almonds.

India

Daal

Also spelled dahl, dal, and dhal.

Yield: 4 servings

1 ½ cups uncooked brown, green, or black lentils, rinsed

3½ cups water

1 small red onion, small dice

¼ cup olive oil

2 Tbs. fresh minced ginger

1 Tbs. curry powder

1 tomato, diced

Juice of one lemon

Salt to taste (about 1½ tsp.)

In a 3-quart saucepan, bring the lentils and water to a boil. Reduce heat to low, cover, and simmer until tender, about 45 minutes.

Drain off water to the point where the water line is just below the lentils. Set aside.

In a 3-quart saucepan, sauté the onion with the oil until tender.

Add ginger and sauté until tender.

Add curry powder.

Add tomato and cook for two minutes.

Add lemon juice.

Add cooked lentils with liquid.

Simmer for 10 minutes.

Add salt to taste.

Fufu Soup Bowl

This is an edible bowl to serve soup in, for example, African Peanut Soup (pg. 32)

Yield: 4 servings

2 yams, peeled and medium dice

Instant mashed potato flakes, about 1 cup

Salt to taste

Pepper to taste

Boil yams until tender. Drain off water.

Mash yams until smooth.

Add instant mashed potatoes until yams are firm enough to be formed into a ball.

Add salt and pepper to taste.

Divide dough into four pieces.

Form each piece into a bowl.

Fill with soup and serve immediately.

Jamaican Rice and Peas

Beans are called peas in Jamaica.

Yield: 4 cups

1¼ cups long grain brown rice, rinsed

14-oz. can unsweetened coconut milk

1½ cups water

15-oz. can kidney beans, drained and rinsed

½ tsp. salt

In a 3-quart saucepan, bring all ingredients to a boil.

Reduce heat to low, cover, and simmer for 45 minutes or until rice is tender.

Jasmine Rice

Yield: 4 cups cooked rice

1½ cups white jasmine rice, rinsed

2 cups water

In a 2-quart saucepan, combine rice and water.

Let sit for 15 minutes.

Bring to a boil, reduce heat to low, cover, and simmer for 15 minutes or until rice is tender.

Mayan Black Beans

Yield: 3 servings

½ cup small diced onion

1 Tbs. vegetable oil

1 Tbs. cocoa powder

2 Tbs. sugar

⅛ tsp. cayenne pepper

15-oz. can black beans, drained and rinsed

1 Tbs. lime juice

2 Tbs. water

Salt to taste

In a 3-quart saucepan, sauté the onion with the oil until tender. Reduce heat to low.

Add cocoa powder, sugar, and cayenne pepper. Cook for 15-30 seconds, stirring constantly.

Add black beans, lime juice, and water.

Over medium heat, heat until hot.

Add salt to taste.

Polenta, firm style

This makes a firm style of polenta, but see the variation for a softer style.

Yield: 4 servings

1 cup vegetable broth

1 cup unsweetened soy milk

½ cup + 2 Tbs. dry polenta (looks like coarse cornmeal)

½ tsp. salt

⅓ cup olive oil for grilling, 3 Tbs. olive oil for baking dish

In a 2-quart saucepan, bring vegetable broth and soy milk to a boil.

Whisk in polenta until mixture thickens, (about one minute) stirring constantly.

Remove from heat, cover, and let sit for 10 minutes.

Pour into an oiled 8-inch × 8-inch baking dish.

Cool in refrigerator for one hour or until set.

Cut into 4 pieces and remove from baking dish.

Preheat griddle to 375°F.

Grill on a lightly oiled griddle until browned on each side.

Variation: Polenta, soft style

Reduce polenta to ⅓ cup.

Refried Beans

Yield: 4 servings

1 cup uncooked pinto beans

5 cups water

1 small onion, small dice

3 Tbs. vegetable oil

1 tsp. garlic powder

1 tsp. onion powder

Salt to taste (about 1¼ tsp.)

In a large pan, combine pinto beans and water. Bring to a boil, reduce heat to low, cover and simmer until tender, about 90–120 minutes (or beans can be soaked overnight to reduce cooking time).

Reserve ½ cup of cooking liquid. Drain off the remaining liquid.

Set beans and reserved liquid aside.

In a large saucepan, sauté the onion with the oil until tender.

Add garlic powder and onion powder. Cook for one minute.

Add beans and reserved cooking liquid.

Heat until hot, stirring constantly.

Add salt to taste.

Leave beans whole or mash.

Roasted Curry Cauliflower

Cauliflower (gobi) is a very popular vegetable in India.

Yield: 4 servings

1 head of cauliflower cut into bite-sized pieces

2 Tbs. olive oil

2 tsp. curry powder

1 tsp. turmeric

¾ tsp. salt

Preheat oven to 475°F.

Place cauliflower in boiling water and boil for five minutes.

Drain off water.

In a large baking dish, toss cauliflower with remaining ingredients.

Bake until browned on the edges, about 15 minutes.

France

Scalloped Potatoes

Yield: 6 servings

5 cups peeled and ⅛-inch sliced russet potatoes (about 4 medium)

1 onion, small dice

⅓ cup vegetable oil

2 Tbs. yeast flakes

1½ tsp. salt

½ tsp. onion powder

¼ tsp. black pepper

¼ tsp. nutmeg

½ cup flour

3½ cups unsweetened soy milk

Preheat oven to 425°F.

Place sliced potatoes in boiling water. Boil just until tender, about 8-10 minutes. Drain and set aside.

In a large pan, sauté the onion with the oil until tender. Add yeast flakes, salt, onion powder, black pepper, and nutmeg. Cook for one minute, stirring constantly.

Add flour and cook for one minute, stirring constantly.

Stir in soy milk and cook until thickened, stirring constantly.

Gently fold in cooked potatoes.

Pour into an oiled 8-inch × 8-inch baking dish.

Bake for 20 minutes.

Spanish Rice

Yield: 4 servings

1 cup brown rice, rinsed

2 cups water

½ onion, small dice

2 Tbs. vegetable oil

1 tsp. chili powder

½ tsp. garlic powder

½ tsp. oregano

½ tsp. sugar

¼ tsp. cumin

¼ cup water

¼ cup tomato paste

Salt to taste (about 1 tsp.)

In a 2-quart saucepan, combine rice and 2 cups of water.

Bring to a boil, reduce heat to low, cover, and simmer for 45 minutes, or until rice is tender.

In a separate 2-quart saucepan, sauté the onion with the oil until tender. Reduce heat to low.

On reduced heat, add chili powder, garlic powder, oregano, sugar, and cumin, and continue to sauté for 1 minute. Add the ¼ cup water and tomato paste.

Add seasoned sautéed onion mix to the cooked rice.

Add salt to taste.

Sushi Rice

Yield: 4 cups

2 cups short grain white rice (sushi rice)

Warm water for rinsing

2½ cups water

¼ cup sugar

¼ cup rice vinegar

1½ tsp. salt

In a 3-quart saucepan, cover rice with warm water. Stir rice around in water. Pour off water. Repeat two more times or until water runs clear.

Add 2½ cups water.

Bring to a boil and stir to make sure rice is not sticking to bottom of pan.

Reduce heat to low, cover and simmer until rice is tender, about 20 minutes.

Place cooked rice in a shallow dish.

Gently fold in sugar, rice vinegar, and salt.

Cool in refrigerator to room temperature before using.

Tempura Vegetables

Serve with Asian Dipping Sauce (pg.286) or soy sauce.

Yield: 6 servings

4 cups bite-sized vegetables (broccoli, onion, cauliflower, squash, eggplant, bell peppers, green beans, and/or mushrooms)

1¼ cups flour

¼ cup cornstarch

1 Tbs. salt

1½ tsp. egg replacer powder

1½ tsp. baking powder

1½ cups unsweetened soy milk

Vegetable oil for frying

Prepare selected vegetables and set aside.

In a large bowl, whisk together the dry ingredients. Whisk in soy milk.

Preheat ½ inch of oil in skillet or recommended amount of oil in a deep fat fryer to 350°F.

In batches, lightly batter vegetables and place in hot oil.

Fry until lightly browned.

Breakfast:

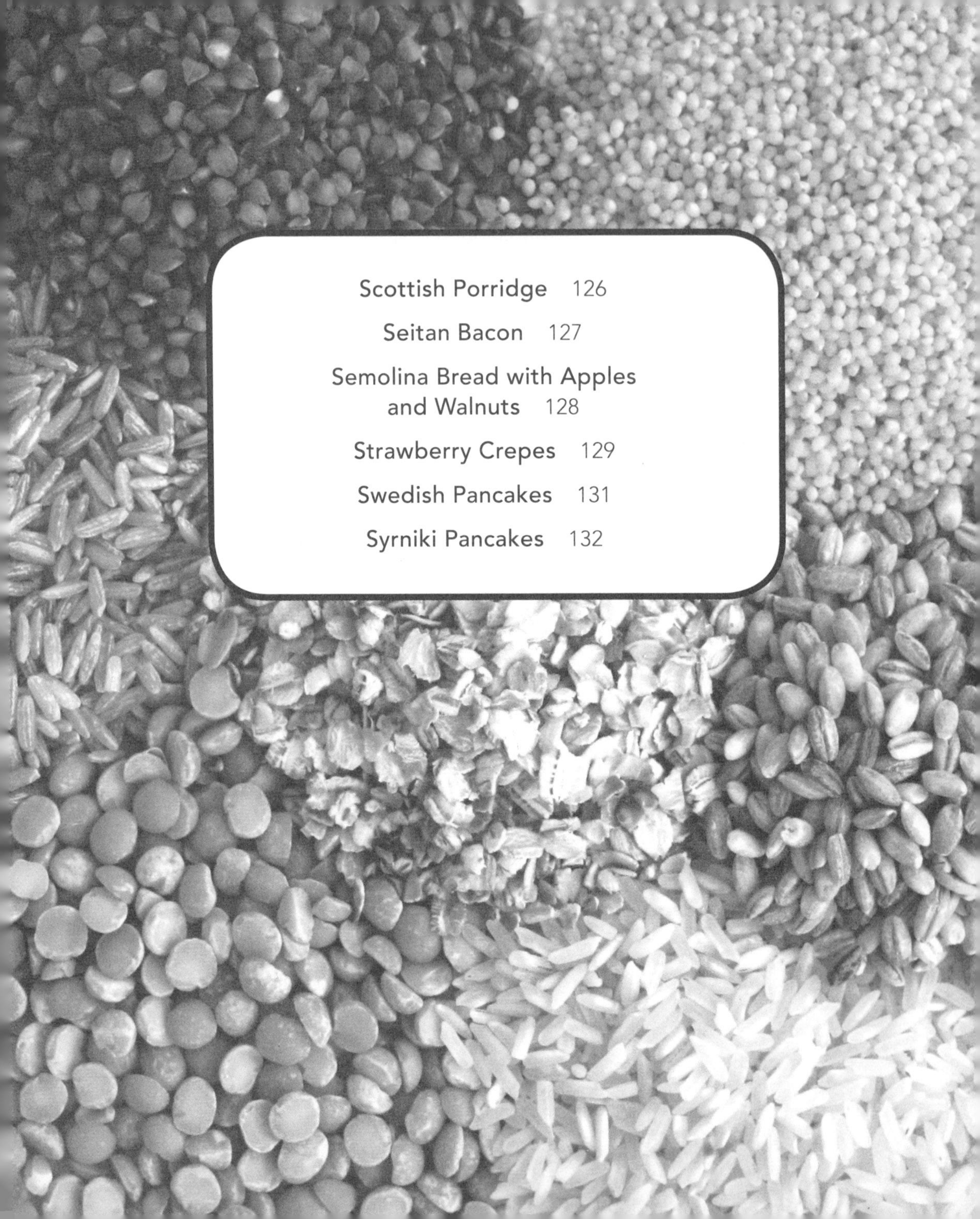

Aebleskivers

Serve dusted with powdered sugar, maple syrup, or jam. You can also fill each aebleskiver with a small piece of apple (or other treat) if preferred.

Yield: 36 (Danish) pancakes

Aebleskiver pan

3 cups flour*

2 Tbs. baking powder

1 Tbs. egg replacer powder

2 tsp. salt

3½ cups soy milk

⅓ cup vegetable oil

1 Tbs. vanilla

1 tsp. apple cider vinegar

Pan spray

** Use part whole wheat flour if you prefer.*

Preheat stovetop aebleskiver pan over medium-low heat. If using an electric aebleskiver pan, preheat following manufacturer's directions.

In a large bowl, whisk together the flour, baking powder, egg replacer powder, and salt.

Whisk in the soy milk, oil, vanilla, and apple cider vinegar.

Pan-spray aebleskiver pan.

Fill each aebleskiver cup with batter until nearly full.

When thin crust has formed on the bottom, take a fork and pull crust up the side of the cup letting the uncooked batter flow down into the cup. Repeat this three more times while rotating the cooked crust clockwise a ¼ turn each time. Stop when there is no uncooked batter left and a ball has formed. Continue to cook ball until batter is fully cooked in the middle.

Repeat with remaining batter, pan-spraying aebleskiver pan each time.

Australia

Aussie Damper, Oven Baked Style

The traditional way to cook this dish is by placing the dough in a Dutch oven and then into a campfire to cook, or by twisting dough around a stick and cooking over a campfire. Add raisins or other dried fruit if preferred. Dampers are sometimes served with Vegemite.

Yield: 6 servings

3 cups flour*

4 tsp. baking powder

1 Tbs. sugar

1½ tsp. salt

1½ cups soy milk

¼ cup vegetable oil

** Use part whole wheat flour if you prefer.*

Preheat oven to 425°F.

In a bowl, whisk together the flour, baking powder, sugar, and salt. Add raisins or dried fruit if preferred.

With a spoon, stir in the soy milk and oil just until moistened.

With moistened hands, form dough into a round loaf.

Place on an oiled baking sheet.

Bake for 15 minutes or until a toothpick inserted in center comes out clean.

Bagels

The iconic New York bagel was brought to the USA by Polish-Jewish immigrants. By 1900 there were 70 bakers in the Lower East Side alone making bagels. In 1907 the Bagels Bakery Union 338 was formed and went on to monopolize bagel production in New York City for decades to come by limiting admission to only sons to ensure recipes were kept secret.

Yield: 6 bagels

1 Tbs. active dry yeast (¼-oz. package)

1 tsp. sugar

¾ cup warm water (110°F)

1¾ cups flour*

1 Tbs. vital wheat gluten flour

1½ tsp. salt

** Use part whole wheat flour if you prefer.*

In a large bowl, whisk together the yeast, sugar, and warm water and let sit 10 minutes.

Add flour, vital wheat gluten flour, and salt.

Knead dough for seven minutes on a floured surface.

Divide dough into six equal-sized dough balls.

Press a hole in the middle of each ball and form into a bagel shape.

Place on a lightly floured surface, cover with a tea towel, and let rise for 30 minutes.

While bagels are rising, bring a large pot of water to a boil, preheat oven to 425°F, and oil one baking sheet.

Boil bagels for two minutes on each side.

Remove from water and place bagels on oiled baking sheet.

Bake for 10 minutes, flip bagels, and bake for 10 more minutes.

Belgian Waffles

Unlike the American version of Belgian waffles, which uses baking powder as a leavening agent, this recipe uses yeast. Traditionally served with sliced strawberries.

Yield: 4 waffles

1 Tbs. active dry yeast (¼-oz. package)

3½ cups warm soy milk (110°F)

1 tsp. sugar

3 cups flour*, divided

1 Tbs. baking powder

½ cup vegetable oil

1 Tbs. vanilla

2 tsp. salt

Pan spray

** Use part whole wheat flour if you prefer.*

In a large bowl add dry yeast. Whisk in warm soy milk and sugar. Let sit for 10 minutes. Whisk in two cups of the flour.

Place dough in a bowl which will accommodate the dough doubling in size. Cover bowl with clear wrap and let sit for one hour on counter or overnight in refrigerator.

Whisk in the remaining one cup of flour, baking powder, oil, vanilla, and salt.

Preheat waffle iron.

Pan-spray top and bottom of hot waffle iron if needed.

Scoop batter onto waffle iron and cook until done, about four minutes.

Repeat until all batter is used.

Biscuits and Gravy

Yield: 12 servings

3 cups Country Gravy (pg. 296)

3¾ cups flour*

5 tsp. baking powder

1½ tsp. salt

1½ cups soy milk

⅔ cup vegetable oil

** Use part whole wheat flour if you prefer.*

Preheat oven to 425°F.

Prepare Country Gravy and set aside.

In a large bowl, whisk together the flour, baking powder, and salt.

With a spoon, stir in the soy milk and oil just until combined.

Turn dough out onto a lightly floured surface.

Roll out to ½-inch thickness.

Cut into 12 pieces.

Place one inch apart on a baking sheet.

Bake for 12 minutes, or until toothpick inserted in center comes out clean.

Split biscuits and top with Country Gravy.

Russia

Blini Buckwheat Pancakes

Traditionally served with sour cream.

Yield: 30 4-inch pancakes

2 cups flour*

1 cup buckwheat flour

2 Tbs. baking powder

1 Tbs. egg replacer powder

2 tsp. salt

3 cups soy milk

⅓ cup vegetable oil

2 Tbs. vanilla

1 Tbs. apple cider vinegar

12 oz. vegan sour cream

** Use part whole wheat flour if you prefer.*

Preheat electric griddle or skillet to 375°F, or put on medium heat if using a stovetop griddle or skillet.

In a large bowl, whisk together the flour, baking powder, egg replacer powder, and salt.

Whisk in the soy milk, oil, vanilla, and vinegar.

Cook pancakes on a lightly oiled griddle, skillet, or frying pan.

Top with sour cream.

Canadian Flapjacks

Quebec, Canada, produces most of the world's supply of maple syrup.

Yield: 24

2 green apples, peeled, cored, and small dice

3 cups flour*

2 Tbs. baking powder

1 Tbs. egg replacer powder

1 tsp. salt

3¼ cup soy milk

2 Tbs. vegetable oil

1 Tbs. lemon juice

1 cup real maple syrup

** Use part whole wheat flour if you prefer.*

Preheat electric griddle or skillet to 350°F, or put on medium-low heat if using a stovetop griddle or skillet.

In a large bowl, combine apples, flour, baking powder, egg replacer powder, and salt.

Whisk in the soy milk, oil, and lemon juice.

Cook flapjacks on a lightly oiled griddle, skillet or frying pan.

Serve with warm maple syrup.

Chilaquiles

Chilaquiles are a Mexican comfort food that often utilizes leftover corn tortillas. Serve with Refried Beans (pg. 96) and/or Spanish Rice (pg. 99) if preferred.

Yield: 2 servings

6 6-inch Corn Tortillas (pg. 230)

3 Tbs. vegetable oil

1 cup Pico De Gallo (pg. 309)

Garnish options:
vegan sour cream, chopped jalapeños, chopped cilantro, vegan jack cheese, avocado, Guacamole (pg.300), chopped onions

Cut tortillas into 1-inch squares.

Heat oil in a large frying pan.

Fry tortillas until crisp, stirring often.

Remove tortillas and place on a plate lined with paper towels.

Add salsa to large frying pan and heat until hot.

Gently stir in tortillas and cook until softened, about two minutes.

Place in a serving dish and garnish as desired.

Chorizo Potato Skillet

Serve with salsa or your favorite hot sauce.

Yield: 6 servings

3 medium potatoes, peeled, large dice

1 onion, small dice

¼ cup vegetable oil

12 oz. vegan chorizo

Salt to taste (about 1 tsp.)

12 oz. vegan jack cheese, shredded

Boil potatoes just until tender, about 15 minutes. Drain and set aside.

In a large skillet, sauté the onion with the oil until tender.

Add potatoes and fry until lightly browned.

Add chorizo and cook until hot.

Add salt to taste.

Top with cheese.

Place in oven with broiler setting on high*.

Broil until cheese is melted.

** If you are using a skillet with a plastic handle, position the skillet so the handle sticks outside of the oven.*

England

Corned Beef Hash

Serve with Country Gravy (pg. 296) or ketchup.

Yield: 3 servings

2 potatoes, peeled and shredded

½ onion, small dice

2 Tbs. vegetable oil

1 cup finely chopped vegan Corned Beef (pg. 151)

Salt and pepper to taste

Place potatoes in a colander. Run cool water over potatoes until water runs clear. Drain off all water. Place shredded potatoes in a clean towel and ring out remaining water. Set potatoes aside.

In a large pan, sauté the onions with the oil until tender.

Add potatoes and corned beef. Fry until crispy, turning as needed.

Add salt and pepper to taste.

Cranberry Almond Scone

Before baking powder was a common kitchen ingredient, these scones were cooked on the grill.

Yield: 12 scones

2½ cups flour*

⅓ cup sugar

2 tsp. baking powder

½ tsp. baking soda

1 tsp. salt

½ cup dried cranberries

½ cup sliced almonds

⅓ cup vegan margarine, melted

6 oz. firm silken tofu (¾ cup)

¾ cup soy milk

1 Tbs. lemon juice

¾ tsp. almond extract

1 Tbs. sugar

** Use part whole wheat flour if you prefer.*

Preheat oven to 425°F.

In a large bowl, whisk together the flour, ⅓ cup sugar, baking powder, baking soda, salt, cranberries, and almonds.

In a blender, blend the margarine, tofu, soy milk, lemon juice, and almond extract.

Add blended ingredients to flour mixture and stir just until combined.

On a floured surface, gently knead dough for one minute.

Form dough into three individual rounded mounds. Cut each mound into four wedges.

Place wedges on an oiled baking sheet.

Sprinkle tops with sugar.

Bake for 17 minutes or until toothpick inserted in center comes out clean.

Crumpets

Crumpets are a cross between a pancake and an English muffin.

Yield: 12

½ cup warm water (110°F)

1 tsp. sugar

1 Tbs. yeast (¼-oz. package)

2½ cups flour*

1¼ tsp. salt

½ tsp. baking soda

1½ cups soy milk

Crumpet rings (optional)

Vegetable oil for grilling

** Use part whole wheat flour if you prefer.*

In a large bowl, whisk together the water, sugar, and yeast and let sit for 10 minutes.

Whisk in flour, salt, baking soda, and soy milk. Cover and let sit at room temperature for one hour.

Preheat electric griddle or skillet to 250°F, or put on low heat if using a stovetop griddle or skillet.

Lightly oil griddle and crumpet rings (if you do not have crumpet rings you can use round metal cookie cutters, or simply cook without any rings like you would pancakes).

Stir batter.

Place rings on griddle. Scoop ⅓ of a cup of batter into each ring.

Grill crumpets until the bubbles on top break and form craters, about 10 minutes.

Remove crumpet rings. Flip over crumpets and cook for one more minute.

English Muffins

Yield: 12

2 Tbs. vegan margarine

½ cup soy milk

½ cup water

1 Tbs. sugar

1 Tbs. yeast (¼-oz. package)

¼ cup vital wheat gluten flour

1 Tbs. salt

2 cups flour*

¼ cup cornmeal

Vegetable oil for grilling

** Use part whole wheat flour if you prefer.*

In a 2-quart saucepan, melt margarine.

Add soy milk, water, and sugar. Heat to 110°F. Be careful this liquid does not continue to heat to over 120°F, which can happen when the container used to heat the liquid continues to heat the liquid after the container is removed from the heat source. Pour into a large bowl.

Whisk in yeast and let sit for 10 minutes.

Whisk in vital wheat gluten flour and salt.

Stir in flour.

On a lightly floured surface, knead for five minutes.

Cover and let rest for five minutes.

Roll out to ½-inch thick.

Cut into 3½-inch rounds, combining scraps to form last couple of rounds.

Place on a cornmeal-dusted baking sheet. Sprinkle top of muffins with cornmeal.

Cover and let rise until doubled in size, about one hour.

English Muffins
(*continued*)

Preheat griddle to 300°F.

Grill on lightly oiled griddle until browned on each side and cooked in the middle, about eight minutes per side.

To serve, split and toast muffins.

Fluffy Pikelets

Yield: 30

3 cups self-rising flour*

1½ Tbs. egg replacer powder

1½ tsp. salt

3¼ cups soy milk

¼ cup melted vegan margarine

2 Tbs. lemon juice

Vegetable oil for grilling

* *If you do not have self-rising flour you can make your own by adding 1½ Tbs. baking powder to three cups of all-purpose flour.*

Preheat electric griddle or skillet to 350°F, or put on medium-low heat if using a stovetop griddle or skillet.

In a large bowl, whisk together the flour, egg replacer powder, and salt.

Whisk in the soy milk, margarine, and lemon juice.

Cook pancakes on a lightly oiled griddle, skillet or frying pan.

USA

Granola

Granola was invented in Dansville, New York, by Dr. James Caleb Jackson. It became popular during the hippie movement of the 1960s.

Yield: Ten ¾-cup servings

4 cups uncooked quick oatmeal

2 cups sliced almonds

1½ cups shredded coconut

¼ cup flax seeds, ground

¼ cup wheat germ

1 tsp. salt

½ cup maple syrup

¼ cup vegetable oil

Preheat oven to 250°F.

In a large bowl, combine dry ingredients.

Stir in maple syrup and oil.

Pour into two 10-inch × 15-inch baking dishes.

Bake for 90 minutes, stirring every 30 minutes. Rotate baking dishes top to bottom after one hour.

Cool completely before storing in an air-tight container.

Lingonberry Drop Muffins

Yield: 12 muffins

2½ cups flour*

½ cup sugar

1 Tbs. baking powder

½ tsp. baking soda

½ tsp. cornstarch

1 tsp. salt

1½ cups soy milk

⅓ cup vegetable oil

2 tsp. vanilla

¾ cup lingonberry jam

** Use part whole wheat flour if you prefer.*

Preheat oven to 400°F.

In a large bowl, whisk together the flour, sugar, baking powder, baking soda, cornstarch, and salt.

Stir in the soy milk, oil, and vanilla just until moistened.

Divide batter between 12 oiled muffin cups.

Push or pipe one Tbs. lingonberry jam into the batter of each muffin, leaving some of the jam exposed on the top of the muffin.

Bake for 20 minutes or until toothpick inserted in center comes out clean.

Switzerland

Muesli

Muesli was invented by Swiss nutritionist Dr. Bircher-Benner. Freshly-grated tart apple is a popular fruit option.

Yield: 4 servings

1½ cups uncooked old-fashioned oatmeal (rolled oats)

½ cup chopped nuts

½ cup dried fruit or 1 cup fresh fruit

2 Tbs. wheat germ

2 Tbs. sunflower seeds

Soy milk, vegan yogurt, or fruit juice to taste

Sweetener to taste

In a bowl, combine rolled oats, nuts, fruit, wheat germ, and sunflower seeds.

Add soy milk, yogurt, or juice a few minutes before eating, or soak overnight in refrigerator.

Add sweetener to taste.

Mushroom and Thyme Omelette

Yield: Six 6-inch omelets

Batter:

1 lb. silken tofu

2 Tbs. olive oil

½ tsp. turmeric

½ tsp. onion powder

½ tsp. garlic powder

¼ tsp. black pepper

¾ tsp. salt

¼ cup + 1 Tbs. cornstarch

¼ cup flour

Filling:

1 cup julienne onions

3 Tbs. olive oil

2 cups sliced mushrooms

½ tsp. fresh thyme leaves, chopped

¼ tsp. salt

In a food processor or blender, mix tofu, 2 Tbs. olive oil, turmeric, onion powder, garlic powder, black pepper, and salt until smooth.

Add cornstarch and flour. Mix just until combined. Set aside.

Sauté onions with oil until caramelized. Add mushrooms and thyme. Sauté until mushrooms are tender and all of its liquid has evaporated.

In a pan-sprayed omelet pan, add 1/6 of the omelet mixture, swirl until desired size, and cook until completely set.

Flip and cook for one more minute.

Fill with 1/6 of the filling.

Fold.

Repeat with remaining batter and filling.

Papa Jalapeño

Serve with salsa or hot sauce.

Yield: 3 servings

4 cups peeled and shredded potatoes

1 fresh jalapeño, chopped

Oil for grilling

Salt to taste

Preheat electric griddle or skillet to 425°F, or put on medium-high heat if using a stovetop griddle or skillet.

Place shredded potatoes in a colander. Run cool water over potatoes until water runs clear.

Drain off excess water. Place potatoes in a towel and squeeze out remaining water.

Combine shredded potatoes with chopped jalapeño.

On a well-oiled griddle, grill potato jalapeño mix until crispy on both sides.

Add salt to taste.

Potato Pancakes

Potato pancakes are the national dish of Belarus. Serve with vegan sour cream for a traditional touch, or serve with apple sauce, jam, maple syrup, or Country Gravy (pg. 296).

Yield: 3 servings

4 cups peeled and shredded potatoes

½ onion, minced

¼ cup soy milk

2 tsp. egg replacer powder

1 tsp. salt

Vegetable oil for grilling

Preheat electric griddle or skillet to 400°F, or put on medium heat if using a stovetop griddle or skillet.

Place shredded potatoes in a colander. Run cool water over potatoes until water runs clear.

Drain excess water. Place potatoes in a towel and squeeze out last remaining water.

In a large bowl, add shredded potatoes, onion, soy milk, egg replacer powder, and salt.

On a well oiled griddle, form mixture into 4-inch patties. Grill until crisp on both sides.

Scottish Porridge

Scottish, steel-cut, and Irish oats are all names for oats cut into 2 or 3 pieces and not rolled flat.

Yield: 4 servings

4 cups water

½ tsp. salt (optional)

1 cup Scottish oatmeal (steel-cut oats)

2 cups cold soy milk, divided*

In a 2-quart saucepan bring water and salt to a boil.

While water is boiling, stir (clockwise*) in oatmeal.

Reduce heat to low and simmer until oats are cooked, about 25-30 minutes, stirring occasionally.

Serve oats with individual bowls filled with ½ cup of cold soymilk per person.

To eat, take a spoonful of oats and then dip it in the soy milk.

** For Scottish good luck.*

Seitan Bacon

Yield: 24 slices

1¼ cups vital wheat gluten flour

2 tsp. onion powder

2 tsp. salt

2 tsp. paprika

½ tsp. black pepper

¾ cup water

¼ cup maple syrup

¼ cup vegetable oil

1 Tbs. molasses

1½ tsp. liquid smoke

Vegetable oil for grilling

Pan spray

Preheat oven to 350°F.

In a large bowl, whisk together the vital wheat gluten flour, onion powder, salt, paprika, and black pepper.

In a separate bowl, whisk together the water, maple syrup, oil, molasses, and liquid smoke.

Combine wet ingredients with dry ingredients just until moistened.

Press into a pan-sprayed 8½-inch × 4½-inch × 2½-inch loaf pan.

Cover with foil and bake for 50 minutes. Remove foil and bake 5 more minutes.

Remove from oven and let cool 10 minutes.

Remove from loaf pan and cut into thin strips.

Grill strips on a 350°F oiled griddle until crispy.

Semolina Bread with Apples and Walnuts

Yield: 9 pieces

1 apple, peeled, cored, and small dice

1 cup semolina flour

¾ cup whole wheat flour

½ cup chopped walnuts

¼ cup brown sugar

2 tsp. baking powder

2 tsp. egg replacer powder

1 tsp. salt

¼ tsp. cinnamon

1 cup soy milk

¼ cup firm silken tofu

⅓ cup vegetable oil

½ tsp. vanilla

Preheat oven to 400°F.

In a large bowl, combine apple, semolina flour, whole wheat flour, walnuts, brown sugar, baking powder, egg replacer powder, salt, and cinnamon.

In a blender, blend soy milk, silken tofu, oil, and vanilla.

Add blended ingredients to the dry mixture and mix just until combined.

Pour batter into an oiled 8-inch × 8-inch baking dish.

Bake for 22 minutes or until toothpick inserted in center comes out clean.

Strawberry Crepes

A very thin pancake traditionally garnished with powdered sugar.

Yield: 4 servings

Filling:

8 oz. vegan cream cheese or sour cream

3 cups sliced strawberries

½ cup sugar

Batter:

2 cups flour

3 Tbs. sugar

2 Tbs. baking powder

1 tsp. salt

12 oz. firm silken tofu

3 cups soy milk

½ cup vegetable oil

1 Tbs. vanilla

Pan spray

Garnish:

2 cups sliced strawberries

¼ cup powdered sugar

Filling:

In a bowl, combine vegan cream cheese or sour cream, strawberries, and sugar. Set aside.

Batter:

In a large bowl, whisk together flour, sugar, baking powder, and salt.

In a blender, blend tofu, soy milk, oil, and vanilla.

Whisk together the blended ingredients with the flour mixture.

Crepes:

Heat a small skillet or crepe pan until medium hot. Pan-spray pan. Pour ⅓ cup of batter in pan. Rotate pan until batter forms a thin layer. Cook until lightly

Strawberry Crepes
(*continued*)

browned. Turn crepe and cook until lightly browned. Remove crepe from pan. Add ¼ cup filling and roll-up.

Repeat until all batter and filling is used.

Garnish crepes with sliced strawberries and powdered sugar.

Swedish Pancakes

These pancakes are served as a dessert in Sweden with lingonberry jam.

Yield: Twenty-four 3-inch pancakes

3 cups soy milk

¼ cup firm silken tofu

2 Tbs. egg replacer powder

1¼ cups flour*

¼ cup sugar

1 tsp. salt

¼ cup vegan margarine, melted

** Use part whole wheat flour if you prefer.*

Preheat electric griddle or skillet to 375°F, or put on medium heat if using a stovetop griddle or skillet.

In a blender, blend soy milk, tofu, and egg replacer powder until smooth.

In a large bowl, combine flour, sugar, and salt.

Combine blended mixture with flour mixture.

Stir in melted margarine.

Cook pancakes on a lightly oiled griddle, skillet or frying pan.

Syrniki Pancakes

Russian "cheese" pancakes. Top your syrniki with sour cream, jam, or apple sauce.

Yield: Thirty 3-inch pancakes

2 cups flour*

½ cup golden raisins

¼ cup sugar

Zest from one lemon, minced

2 Tbs. baking powder

1 tsp. salt

2½ cups soy milk

8 oz. vegan cream cheese

Juice of one lemon

** Use part whole wheat flour if you prefer.*

Preheat electric griddle or skillet to 350°F, or put on medium-low heat if using a stovetop griddle or skillet.

In a large bowl, whisk together the flour, raisins, sugar, lemon zest, baking powder, and salt.

In a blender, blend soy milk, cream cheese, and lemon juice until smooth.

Whisk together the blended mixture with the flour mixture.

Cook pancakes on a lightly oiled griddle, skillet, or frying pan.

Entrees:

Asian Noodle Bowl with Edamame Jade Pesto

Yield: 5 servings

1¾ cups Edamame Jade Pesto Sauce (pg. 298)

12 oz. refrigerated precooked yakisoba noodles

1 lb. firm tofu, medium dice

1 Tbs. vegetable oil

½ tsp. paprika

½ tsp. onion powder

¼ tsp. salt

Garnish options: shredded yam, shredded carrot, diced green onion, shredded purple and/or green cabbage, toasted sliced almonds and/or chopped cashews, chopped cilantro or basil, roasted garlic, roasted or fresh julienned red onions, Roasted Edamame (pg. 336), vegan sriracha sauce, sweet chili sauce, soy sauce

Prepare Edamame Jade Pesto Sauce and set aside.

Grill tofu with oil until lightly crisp. Add paprika, onion powder, and salt. Set aside.

Boil yakisoba noodles until hot. Drain.

To serve, place yakisoba noodles in a bowl and top with Jade Pesto Sauce and tofu.

Garnish as desired.

Barbecue Ribz

Great with Cheesy Brown Rice, (pg. 86).

Yield: 4 servings

¾ cup Barbecue Sauce (pg. 288)

1¼ cups vital wheat gluten flour

1 Tbs. paprika

1 tsp. onion powder

1 tsp. salt

1 cup water

6 Tbs. vegetable oil, divided

½ tsp. liquid smoke

Pan spray

Preheat oven to 325°F.

Prepare Barbecue Sauce and set aside.

In a large bowl, whisk together vital wheat gluten flour, paprika, onion powder, and salt.

In a separate bowl, whisk together water, three Tbs. of the oil, and liquid smoke.

Combine wet ingredients with dry ingredients just until moistened.

Press into a pan-sprayed 8-inch × 8-inch baking dish.

Bake for 40 minutes.

Remove from oven and cut into strips.

In a large frying pan, sauté the strips with the remaining 3 Tbs. of oil until crispy, stirring often.

Add Barbecue Sauce and cook until hot.

Basil Tofu Stir Fry

Yield: 4 servings

1¾ cups Asian Dipping Sauce (pg. 286) or your favorite teriyaki sauce

16 oz. extra firm tofu, large dice

¼ cup cornstarch

½ tsp. salt

⅓ cup vegetable oil

1 red bell pepper, large dice

1 yellow bell pepper, large dice

1 medium sweet onion, large dice

¼ cup minced fresh ginger

4 Thai bird chilies, small dice (you can substitute with serrano or jalapeño chilies)

1 bunch fresh Thai basil or sweet basil, stems removed and leaves lightly chopped

Prepare Asian Dipping Sauce and set aside.

Toss tofu with cornstarch and salt.

In a large pan, sauté the tofu with the oil until crispy on all sides.

Remove tofu from pan and use the same oil to sauté the vegetables.

Sauté the red bell pepper, yellow bell pepper, sweet onion, ginger, and chilies until tender.

Add prepared tofu to vegetables. Sauté for one minute.

Add sauce and basil.

Cook until basil wilts.

Black Lentil Daal

Lentils were placed in Egyptian tombs as far back as 2400 B.C. Serve with Pita (pg. 237) or Naan (pg. 236) if preferred.

Yield: 6 servings

4 cups cooked Brown Rice (pg. 85)

1¼ cups black beluga lentils

½ red onion, minced

¼ cup olive oil

¼ cup fresh minced ginger

1½ tsp. curry powder

1 tsp. cumin

¼ tsp. cayenne pepper (optional)

2 tomatoes, medium dice

¼ cup lemon juice

Salt to taste (about 2 tsp.)

Garnish options:
chopped red onions,
chopped cilantro or mint,
lemon or lime wedges,
roasted jalapeño,
Raita (pg. 312)

Prepare rice and set aside.

In a large pot, boil lentils until tender, about 45 minutes.

Drain off water to the point where the water line is just below the lentils and set lentils and remaining water aside.

In a 3-quart saucepan, sauté the onion with the oil until tender.

Add ginger and cook until tender.

Add curry powder, cumin, cayenne pepper, and tomatoes. Sauté for one minute.

Add cooked lentils with its remaining water.

Add lemon juice.

Bring to a boil. Reduce heat to low and simmer for 10 minutes, stirring frequently.

Add salt to taste.

Serve over rice.

Garnish as desired.

Blackened Tofu

Great with Hush Puppies (pg. 16).

Yield: 4 servings

½ cup Spicy Orange Sauce (pg. 313)

16 oz. extra firm tofu

¼ cup Cajun Seasoning*

Vegetable oil for grilling

Preheat oven to 350°F.

Prepare Spicy Orange Sauce and set aside.

Cut tofu into four slabs.

Rub Cajun Seasoning on all sides of tofu.

Preheat electric griddle or skillet to 425°F, or put on medium-high heat setting on your stove if using a stovetop griddle or skillet.

On a well oiled griddle, grill tofu on both sides until crisp.

Place tofu in baking dish.

Bake for 30 minutes.

Serve with dipping sauce on the side.

*** Cajun Seasoning**

Yield: ¼ cup

2 Tbs. paprika

2 tsp. garlic powder

2 tsp. salt

1 tsp. onion powder

1 tsp. cayenne pepper

In a small bowl, combine all ingredients.

Black-eyed Peas and Mushrooms

There are over 13,000 species of pulses/legumes (pulses are the seeds of a legume plant). Serve with Pita (pg. 237) or Naan (pg. 236) if preferred.

Yield: 5 servings

4 cups cooked Brown Rice (pg. 85)

1 medium red onion, small dice

¼ cup vegetable oil

1½ pounds mushrooms, sliced

¼ cup minced fresh ginger

1 Tbs. paprika

½ tsp. red pepper flakes (optional)

2 tomatoes, medium dice

15-oz. can black-eyed peas, drained and rinsed

2 Tbs. lemon juice

Salt to taste (about 1½ tsp.)

Prepare rice and set aside.

In a large pan, sauté the onion with the oil until tender.

Add mushrooms and ginger. Sauté until mushrooms are tender. Reduce heat to medium-low.

Add paprika, red pepper flakes, tomatoes, black-eyed peas, and lemon juice.

Simmer for 10 minutes.

Add salt to taste.

Serve over rice.

Broccoli Quiche

Yield: Two 9-inch pies

2 9-inch single precooked Pie Crusts (pg. 334)

6 cups small diced broccoli (floweretts and stems)

1 onion, small dice

¼ cup vegetable oil

16 oz. extra firm tofu, crumbled

½ cup soy milk

¼ cup nutritional yeast flakes

2 Tbs. cornstarch

2 Tbs. flour

2 tsp. salt

⅛ tsp. black pepper

10 oz. vegan jack cheese, shredded

Prepare precooked pie crusts.

Reduce oven temperature to 350°F.

Sauté the broccoli and onion with the oil until tender. Set aside.

In a food processor, combine tofu, soy milk, nutritional yeast flakes, cornstarch, flour, salt, and pepper until smooth. Transfer to a large bowl.

Add sautéed vegetables and cheese.

Transfer to prepared baked pie crusts.

Bake for 45 minutes.

California Sushi Roll

Yield: 8 servings

4 cups cooked and cooled Sushi Rice (pg. 100)

8 7½-inch X 4-inch sheets of nori

8 tsp. black or white sesame seeds, toasted*

2 ripe avocadoes, peeled, pitted, and cut in 12 strips each

1 cucumber, peeled, seeded, and cut into 8 long strips

Garnish options:
pickled ginger, wasabi, soy sauce, rice vinegar

Prepare Sushi Rice and set aside.

Place one nori sheet (shiny side down) on a piece of clear wrap, with long edge of nori horizontal to edge of counter.

Moisten hands with water. Form ½ cup of rice into a lightly packed cylinder about the same length of the long side of the nori sheet.

Place rice on nori and spread out until it covers the nori.

Sprinkle rice with one tsp. sesame seeds.

Pick nori sheet and rice up and flip it over so the rice is now touching the clear wrap.

Place three avocado strips and one cucumber strip lengthwise down the middle.

Using the clear wrap, firmly roll up the sushi. Use a sushi mat under the clear wrap to create a tighter wrap if preferred.

With a sharp knife, use a gentle sawing motion to cut the sushi roll into 6 pieces, cleaning knife with a wet towel as needed.

Repeat seven more times with remaining ingredients.

California Sushi Roll
(*continued*)

***Toasted Sesame Seeds**

sesame seeds	Preheat oven to 350°F. Spread sesame seeds on a baking sheet. Bake for five to seven minutes or until lightly browned (watch closely as they can go from toasted to burnt quickly).

Cannelloni / Manicotti with Spinach and Ricotta

Cannelloni should not be confused with manicotti, which is an Italian crepe. When shopping for cannelloni pasta you can use the often-mislabeled "manicotti" tube pasta.

Yield: 6

2 cups Marinara Sauce (pg. 303)

1¼ cups vegan Ricotta Cheese (pg. 335)

10 oz. frozen chopped spinach, thawed

½ onion, minced

1 Tbs. vegetable oil

2 tsp. onion powder

6 cannelloni /manicotti noodles (about 4 oz.)

Preheat oven to 325°F.

Prepare Marinara Sauce and set aside.

Prepare Ricotta Cheese, place in a pastry bag, and set aside.

Squeeze out excess water from spinach. Set aside spinach.

In a 2-quart saucepan, sauté the onion with the oil until tender.

In a large bowl, combine ricotta cheese, spinach, sautéed onion, and onion powder.

Boil cannelloni according to package directions, being careful not to overcook. Strain off water and cool cannelloni with cold water.

Place half of the Marinara Sauce lengthwise down the middle of a 9-inch × 13-inch baking dish.

Pipe ricotta cheese mixture into cannelloni.

Arrange filled cannelloni on top of the marinara.

Put remaining Marinara Sauce on top of the cannelloni, covering it completely.

Bake, covered, for 25 minutes.

Chana Masala

Serve with Pita (pg. 237) or Naan (pg. 236) if preferred.

Yield: 6 servings

4 cups cooked Brown Rice (pg. 85)

1 small red onion, small dice

3 Tbs. olive oil

¼ cup minced fresh ginger

1 tsp. cumin powder

1 tsp. garam masala

1 tsp. curry powder

¼ tsp. cayenne (optional)

2 12-oz. cans garbanzo beans, drained and rinsed

2 tomatoes, medium dice

Juice of 1 lemon (¼ cup)

1 cup water

Salt to taste (about 1½ tsp.)

Garnish options:
Raita (pg. 312), chopped red onions, chopped cilantro, chopped jalapeños, lemon wedges

Prepare rice and set aside.

In a 3-quart saucepan, sauté the onion with the oil until tender.

Add ginger and sauté until tender.

Reduce heat to medium-low.

Add cumin, garam masala, curry, and cayenne. Sauté for one minute.

Add garbanzos, tomatoes, lemon juice, and water.

Chana Masala
(*continued*)

Bring to a boil. Reduce heat to low and simmer for 15 minutes, stirring frequently.

Add salt to taste.

Serve over rice.

Garnish as desired.

Chili Rellenos

Yield: 12-14

2 cups Enchilada Sauce (pg. 299)

1¼ cups vegan Ricotta Cheese (pg. 335)

3 7-oz. cans whole green chilies, drained

Batter:

1¼ cups flour

¼ cup cornstarch

1 Tbs. salt

1½ tsp. baking powder

1¼ cups soy milk

Vegetable oil for frying

Prepare Enchilada Sauce and set aside.

Prepare Ricotta Cheese and set aside.

Remove and discard any blackened bits on peppers.

Fill chilies with ricotta cheese (use a pastry bag if you have one) and set aside.

Batter:

In a large bowl whisk together the flour, cornstarch, salt, and baking powder. Whisk in the soy milk.

Add ¼-inch of oil to a large skillet.

Heat oil to 350°F.

Lightly batter each stuffed chili and place in hot oil.

Cook rellenos until golden brown on each side.

Top with Enchilada Sauce just before serving.

Chix'n Cacciatore

Cacciatore means "hunter" in Italian…
I would like to think "gatherer" in vegan.

Yield: 4 servings

8 oz. uncooked penne pasta

½ onion, julienne cut

1 green bell pepper, julienne cut

3 Tbs. olive oil

2½ cups sliced mushrooms (½ lb.)

½ tsp. basil

½ tsp. oregano

½ tsp. onion powder

½ tsp. garlic powder

¼ tsp. thyme

¼ tsp. black pepper

3 Tbs. red wine vinegar

14-oz. can fire roasted diced tomatoes

6 oz. vegan chix'n strips

Salt to taste (about 2 tsp.)

Garnish options:
chopped basil or oregano

Cook pasta according to directions. Drain and set aside.

In a large pan, sauté the onion and pepper with the olive oil until tender.

Add mushrooms and continue to sauté until mushrooms are tender.

Add basil, oregano, onion powder, garlic powder, thyme, and black pepper. Sauté for one minute.

Add red wine vinegar and tomatoes and cook for one minute.

Add vegan chicken strips and cook until hot.

Add salt to taste.

Toss with cooked pasta.

Garnish as desired.

Chix'n Marinara

Top with vegan Parmesan Cheese (pg. 330) or freshly chopped basil.

Yield: 6 servings

1 onion, small dice

3 Tbs. olive oil

1 Tbs. basil

2 tsp. onion powder

2 tsp. oregano

1 tsp. sugar

28-oz. can crushed tomatoes

6-oz. can tomato paste

Salt to taste (about 2 tsp.)

16 oz. uncooked pasta

6 breaded vegan chix'n patties

Preheat oven to 350°F.

In a 3-quart saucepan, sauté the onion with the oil until tender.

Add the basil, onion powder, oregano, and sugar and sauté for one minute.

Add crushed tomatoes and tomato paste.

Add salt to taste.

Cover and simmer until needed.

Cook pasta according to package directions. Drain and set aside.

On a baking sheet, heat chix'n patties according to package instructions.

To serve, place an individual serving of pasta on a plate and top with a chix'n patty and sauce.

Corned Beef

Yield: Enough to make 8 Rueben Sandwiches (pg. 192)

- **1¼ cups vital wheat gluten flour**
- **1 Tbs. onion powder**
- **1 Tbs. paprika**
- **1 Tbs. whole ground fennel seed**
- **1 Tbs. whole ground caraway seed**
- **2 tsp. salt**
- **¼ tsp. ground cloves**
- **¼ tsp. ground black pepper**
- **1 cup water**
- **3 Tbs. vegetable oil**
- **1 Tbs. molasses**
- **Cheesecloth (one double-thick 24-inch by 16-inch piece)**
- **2 6-inch pieces of string**

Put 12 cups of water on to boil to be used in step eight.

In a large bowl, whisk together the gluten flour, onion powder, paprika, fennel, caraway, salt, cloves, and black pepper.

In a separate bowl, whisk together the water, oil, and molasses.

Combine wet ingredients with dry ingredients.

Form into a flat, rectangular loaf about 1-inch thick.

Place loaf on 16-inch edge of cheesecloth and wrap the cheesecloth around the loaf (like a candy wrapper).

Tie each end with a piece of string.

Place loaf in gently boiling water.

Cover and simmer for 45 minutes.

Remove roast from water and remove cheesecloth.

England and Ireland

Cottage Pie

At one time Cottage Pie was made with a top and bottom potato crust. It is also known as Shepherd's Pie.

Yield: 6 servings

4 cups mashed potatoes

3 carrots, peeled, medium dice

4 stalks celery, medium dice

1 onion, small dice

¼ cup vegetable oil

¼ cup flour

12 oz. vegan soy ground, or 14-oz. can kidney beans, drained and rinsed

6-oz. can tomato paste

1 cup frozen corn

3 cups vegetable broth

Salt to taste (about 2 tsp.)

Pepper to taste (about ½ tsp.)

Prepare mashed potatoes and set aside.

Preheat oven to 375°F.

In a large saucepan, sauté the carrots, celery, and onion with the oil until tender.

Add flour and cook for one minute.

Add remaining ingredients except mashed potatoes, salt, and pepper. Heat until hot.

Add salt and pepper to taste.

Pour into a 9-inch × 13-inch baking dish.

Top with mashed potatoes.

Bake for 20 minutes.

Eggplant Parmesan

Yield: 3 servings

¾ cup vegan Parmesan (pg. 330)

2 cups Marinara Sauce (pg. 303)

8 oz. uncooked fettuccini noodles

1 large eggplant peeled and cut into 6 wheels

½ cup flour

½ cup soy milk

Vegetable oil for grilling

Garnish options: chopped basil, chopped oregano

Prepare Parmesan and set aside.

Prepare Marinara Sauce and set aside.

On a shallow plate or pie dish, combine flour with parmesan cheese.

In a second shallow plate or pie dish add soy milk.

Dredge eggplant wheels in flour mixture, dredge in soy milk, and dredge a second time in the flour mixture.

In a frying pan, grill eggplant in oil until crisp on each side.

While frying eggplant, prepare fettuccini according to package directions.

Reheat Marinara Sauce.

Serve grilled eggplant with Marinara Sauce and fettuccini.

Garnish as desired.

India

Eggplant with Tamarind

Tamarind, which is widely grown in India, is a fruit pod also known as an "Indian Date." Serve with Pita (pg. 237) or Naan (pg. 236) if preferred.

Yield: 4 servings

Garnish options:
diced red onions, chopped cilantro, chopped jalapeño, lime wedges, Raita (pg. 312)

4 cups cooked Brown Rice (pg. 85)

1 red onion, small dice

¼ cup olive oil

4 cups peeled and large diced eggplant (India eggplant if available)

1 tsp. cumin powder

1 tsp. turmeric

⅛ tsp. cayenne pepper (optional)

15-oz. can lentils with liquid

15-oz. can diced tomatoes with liquid

¼ cup tamarind paste

Salt to taste (about 1½ tsp.)

Prepare rice and set aside.

In a large pan, sauce onion with oil until tender.

Add eggplant and sauté just until tender.

Add cumin, turmeric, and cayenne pepper. Cook for one minute.

Add lentils with liquid, tomatoes with liquid, and tamarind.

Bring to a boil, reduce heat to low, and simmer for 10 minutes.

Add salt to taste.

Serve over rice.

Empanadas

Serve with Pico De Gallo (pg. 309) or Chipotle Dipping Sauce (pg. 292).

Yield: 8 baked* or fried Empanadas**

1 batch Basic Dough (pg. 324)

1 onion, small dice

3 Tbs. vegetable oil

15-oz. can hominy, drained and rinsed

15-oz. can black beans, drained and rinsed

7-oz. can diced green chilies

1 tsp. onion powder

1 tsp. chili powder

Salt to taste (about 1½ tsp.)

Vegetable oil for frying or baking

Prepare Basic Dough, cover, and set aside.

In a large pan, sauté the onion with the oil until tender.

Add hominy, black beans, green chilies, onion powder, and chili powder. Cook for one minute.

Add salt to taste and set aside.

Divide basic dough into eight pieces.

Roll one piece of dough into a 6-inch round.

Place ⅓ cup of filling in middle of dough round.

Fold the dough over, forming a semi-circle. Press the edges together with the tines of a fork.

Repeat with remaining dough and filling.

Choose either the baked or fried method below:

**Baked method:*
Preheat oven to 425°F. Place Empanadas in an oiled baking dish. Brush with oil. Bake for 20 minutes.

***Fried method:*
Preheat ¼-inch of oil in a skillet or recommended amount of oil in a deep fat fryer to 350°F. Fry Empanadas until golden brown on each side, turning as necessary.

Mexico

Enchiladas Papas

Enchiladas were originally made by the Aztecs.
The word enchilada means "dipped in chili."
Original enchiladas were tortillas dipped in sauce.

Yield: 18 enchiladas

2½ cups Enchilada Sauce (pg. 299)

8 cups small diced red potatoes (about 2½ lbs.)

1 onion, small dice

1 cup corn

1 Tbs. chili powder

1 tsp. onion powder

2 tsp. salt

¼ cup vegetable oil

12 oz. vegan jack cheese, shredded

18 6-inch Corn Tortillas (pg. 230)

Vegetable oil for brushing

Prepare Enchilada Sauce and set aside.

Boil potatoes until soft but not mushy.

Preheat oven to 450°F.

In a large baking dish, combine potatoes, onion, corn, chili powder, onion powder, salt, and vegetable oil.

Bake for 20 minutes.

Reduce heat to 350°F.

Place roasted potato mixture in a large bowl and add cheese while potatoes are still hot.

Cover the bottom of a large baking dish with one cup Enchilada Sauce and set aside.

Soften tortillas by lightly brushing each tortilla with oil. Place oiled tortillas on a warm griddle, or microwave until softened.

Place ¼ cup of filling in each softened tortilla and roll up.

Place filled enchiladas in the baking dish.

Top enchiladas with remaining sauce.

Cover and bake for 15 minutes.

English Pasty

A savory hand-held stuffed pastry which was served to English miners.

Yield: 8

2 cups small diced red potatoes

1 small onion, small dice

1 rutabaga*, peeled and small dice

3 Tbs. vegetable oil

1 cup peas

1 tsp. onion powder

1 tsp. garlic powder

½ tsp. black pepper

2 Tbs. stone ground mustard

15-oz. can garbanzo beans, drained and rinsed

Salt to taste

1 batch Basic Dough (pg. 324)

Vegetable oil for brushing

** Substitute rutabaga with parsnips, carrots, or other root vegetables if preferred*

In a large pan, sauté the potatoes, onion, and rutabaga with the oil until tender.

Add peas, onion powder, garlic powder, black pepper, stone ground mustard, and garbanzo beans.

Add salt to taste.

Chill filling.

Prepare Basic Dough.

Divide dough into eight pieces.

Divide filling into eight portions.

Roll one piece of dough into a 6-inch round.

English Pastry
(*continued*)

Place one portion of filling in middle of dough round.

Fold the dough over, forming a semi-circle. Press the edges together with the tines of a fork.

Place pasty in an oiled baking dish.

Repeat with remaining dough and filling.

Brush tops of pasties with oil.

Preheat oven to 425°F.

Bake for 20 minutes.

Brush with oil.

Fajitas

A traditional "Tex-Mex" dish prepared by cowboys on the Texas-Mexico border in the 1930s. Serve with shredded lettuce, Guacamole (pg. 300), vegan sour cream, and/or salsa.

Yield: 6 servings

1¼ cups vital wheat gluten flour

1 Tbs. paprika

1 tsp. chili powder

1 tsp. onion powder

1 tsp. garlic powder

½ tsp. ground cumin

1½ tsp. salt

1 cup water

2 Tbs. vegetable oil

1 red bell pepper, julienne cut

1 green bell pepper, julienne cut

1 onion, julienne cut

3 Tbs. vegetable oil

12 small Flour Tortillas (pg. 234)

Pan spray

Preheat oven to 325°F.

In a large bowl whisk together the vital wheat gluten flour, paprika, chili powder, onion powder, garlic powder, cumin, and salt.

Add water and two Tbs. oil and stir just until combined.

Press dough into a pan-sprayed 8-inch × 8-inch baking dish.

Bake 40 minutes.

Remove seitan from baking dish and cut into ¼-inch × 3-inch strips.

In a large frying pan, sauté the seitan strips, red pepper, green pepper, and onion with the 3 Tbs. of oil until vegetables are tender.

Warm tortillas.

Fill open-faced tortillas with fajita mix and favorite condiments.

Falafel

Garbanzo beans can be substituted with fava beans.

Yield: 6 servings

- **1 cup Tzatziki Sauce (pg. 321)**
- **2 15-oz. cans garbanzo or fava beans, drained and rinsed**
- **2 Tbs. olive oil**
- **⅓ cup lemon juice**
- **½ cup chopped parsley**
- **1 Tbs. ground cumin**
- **2 tsp. garlic powder***
- **2 tsp. salt**
- **½ tsp. baking powder**
- **⅛ tsp. cayenne pepper (optional)**
- **¾ cup flour****
- **Vegetable oil for frying**
- **6 Pitas (pg. 237), grilled**

Filling options:
shredded lettuce, diced tomato, thinly sliced red onion, tahini sauce

Prepare Tzatziki Sauce and set aside.

In a food processor, process the garbanzo beans, 2 Tbs. oil, lemon juice, parsley, cumin, garlic, salt, baking powder, and cayenne pepper until smooth.

Transfer mixture to a bowl and stir in flour.

Preheat ½-inch of oil in skillet or recommended amount of oil in a deep fat fryer to 350°F.

Carefully lower walnut-sized scoops of the falafel dough into the hot oil.

Fry falafel until browned on all sides and no longer doughy in the middle, about four minutes.

Serve falafel open-faced on pita

Fill as desired.

**Use 4 roasted garlic cloves if you prefer.*

***Use half garbanzo bean flour if available.*

Falafel Dogs

Like a corndog but made with falafel batter instead of corn batter.

Yield: 6 baked* or fried Falafel Dogs**

6 vegan hot dogs

15-oz. can garbanzo beans, drained and rinsed

¼ cup lemon juice

1 Tbs. vegetable oil

1 tsp. ground cumin

1 tsp. garlic powder

¾ tsp. salt

¼ tsp. baking powder

¾ cup flour

Vegetable oil for frying or baking

Dipping sauce options: Chipotle Dipping Sauce (pg. 292), hot sauce, Tzatziki Sauce (pg. 321), yellow mustard, ketchup

In a food processor, process the garbanzo beans, lemon juice, oil, cumin, garlic powder, salt and baking powder until smooth.

Add flour and continue to process until smooth.

Divide dough into six portions.

On a lightly floured surface, press out each piece of dough to 4-inches × 5-inches. Place one hot dog in the middle of each piece of dough and form dough around hot dog. Roll until edges are smooth.

Choose either the baked or fried method below:

**Baked method:*
Preheat oven to 450°F. Place Falafel Dogs on an oiled baking sheet, brush with oil, and bake for 15 minutes.

***Fried method:*
Preheat ¼-inch of oil in a skillet or recommended amount of oil in a deep fat fryer to 350°F. Fry Falafel Dogs until golden brown on each side, turning as necessary.

Fettuccini Alfredo

Named by Alfredo di Lello, an Italian restaurateur.

Yield: 4 servings

½ onion, minced

⅓ cup olive oil

1 Tbs. basil

2 tsp. oregano

2 tsp. sugar

1 tsp. garlic powder

⅛ tsp. black pepper

½ cup flour

¼ cup nutritional yeast flakes

4 cups plain unsweetened soy milk

Salt to taste (about 2 tsp.)

12 oz. uncooked fettuccini

In a 3-quart saucepan, sauté the onion with the oil until tender.

Add basil, oregano, sugar, garlic powder, black pepper, and flour and sauté for one minute.

Stir in yeast flakes.

Whisk in soy milk.

Cook until hot and thickened, stirring constantly.

Add salt to taste.

Turn heat to low and keep sauce warm until pasta is cooked.

Cook pasta according to package directions. Drain and rinse with hot tap water.

Serve sauce over pasta.

Focaccia Pizza

Yield: 4 servings

9-inch x 13-inch cooked Focaccia Bread (pg. 235)

1 large sweet onion, small dice

2 Tbs. olive oil

½ cup Pizza Sauce (pg. 310)

8 oz. vegan pepperoni

10 oz. vegan mozzarella, shredded

Prepare Focaccia Bread and set aside.

Sauté the onion with the oil until tender.

Preheat oven broiler setting to high

Top focaccia with Pizza Sauce, pepperoni, onions, and cheese.

Place pizza on middle rack in oven.

Broil until cheese is melted, about two minutes.

Fried Rice

Yield: 4 servings

4 cups cooked Brown Rice (pg. 85)

4 cups total assorted vegetables:

chopped bok choy, chopped napa cabbage, thin bias-cut carrots, thin bias-cut celery, julienne cut onions, julienne cut bell pepper, julienne cut snow peas, cut baby corn, sliced water chestnuts, minced ginger, sliced mushrooms, peas, shelled edamame

7 oz. tempeh bacon, small dice

1 Tbs. toasted sesame oil

2 Tbs. vegetable oil

Soy sauce to taste

Prepare rice and set aside.

In a large pan, sauté the vegetables with the oils until tender.

Add tempeh and cook until hot.

Add cooked rice.

Add soy sauce to taste.

Gnocchi with Roasted Garlic Pesto Sauce

"Gnocchi" is the Italian word for dumpling.

Yield: 4 servings

15 peeled cloves of garlic (one whole garlic bulb)

½ cup olive oil

¼ cup pine nuts or walnuts

¾ tsp. salt

2 bunches basil, stemmed

16 oz. vegan gnocchi

Preheat oven to 375°F.

In a small baking dish, toss garlic with olive oil.

Bake for 20 minutes.

Cool garlic and oil for 30 minutes in the refrigerator.

In a food processor, combine roasted garlic and oil, pine nuts or walnuts, and salt until smooth.

Add basil and pulse blade just until smooth.

Cook gnocchi according to package directions.

Strain gnocchi and toss with prepared Pesto Sauce.

Place in a sauté pan and heat just until hot.

Greece

Gyro Sandwich

Serve with Cucumber Salad (pg. 59) and/or Quinoa Tabbouleh Salad (pg. 69)

Yield: 6 servings

1¼ cups vital wheat gluten flour

1 Tbs. oregano

1 Tbs. garlic powder

2 tsp. paprika

2 tsp. salt

½ tsp. black pepper

1 cup water

3 Tbs. olive oil

3 Tbs. vegetable oil for grilling

6 Pitas (pg. 237)

Pan spray

Filling and Sauce options: shredded lettuce, diced tomato, thinly sliced red onion, Tzatziki Sauce (pg. 321), tahini sauce

Preheat oven to 325°F.

In a large bowl combine flour, oregano, garlic powder, paprika, salt, and black pepper.

Stir in water and oil just until combined.

Press into an 8-inch × 8-inch pan-sprayed baking dish.

Bake for 40 minutes.

Remove seitan from pan and cut into ¼-inch × 3-inch strips.

In a frying pan, lightly grill strips with vegetable oil.

Warm pitas in oven or microwave.

Place gyro strips open-faced on pita.

Add desired fillings and sauce.

Holiday "Turkey"

Yield: 16 servings

1 gallon water

5 cups vital wheat gluten flour

1 cup nutritional yeast flakes

2 tsp. thyme

2 Tbs. onion powder

2 Tbs. salt

4 cups vegetable broth

⅓ cup vegetable oil

2 Tbs. soy sauce

Cheesecloth (one double thick 24-inch X 16-inch piece)

4 10-inch pieces of string

1 sheet ready-to-bake vegan puff pastry, thawed

2 Tbs. ketchup

1 Tbs. water

1 tsp. thyme

In a large pot, bring one gallon of water to a low boil.

In a large bowl, whisk together the vital wheat gluten flour, yeast flakes, 2 tsp. thyme, onion powder, and salt.

Add the vegetable broth, oil, and soy sauce. Stir just until combined.

Form into a loaf shape.

Place loaf on cheesecloth and roll up (not too tight).

Tie each end with a piece of string and tie two additional pieces of sting ⅓ in from each end.

Place in low-boiling water.

Holiday "Turkey"
(*continued*)

Cover pot with lid and cook for one hour and 45 minutes.

Remove loaf from water and remove cheesecloth.

Preheat oven to 400°F.

Roll out puff pastry so that it will cover the loaf.

Cover loaf with puff pastry, tucking edges underneath.

Combine the ketchup, water, and one tsp. thyme.

Brush puff pastry with ketchup mixture.

Bake loaf for 25 minutes.

Italian Meatball Sub

Yield: 6

2 cups Marinara Sauce (pg. 303)

Meatballs:

1¼ cups vital wheat gluten flour

1 Tbs. paprika

1½ tsp. onion powder

1½ tsp. garlic powder

1½ tsp. basil

1½ tsp. oregano

¼ tsp. ground black pepper

1½ tsp. salt

¾ cup water

¼ cup vegetable oil

Subs:

¼ cup vegetable oil

6 sub rolls sliced ¾ of the way through lengthwise (like a hot dog bun)

5 oz. shredded vegan mozzarella or jack cheese

Prepare Marinara Sauce and set aside.

Meatballs:

In a large bowl, whisk together the vital wheat gluten flour, paprika, onion powder, garlic powder, basil, oregano, black pepper, and salt. Add water and the ¼ cup of oil all at once and stir until well combined.

Form dough into walnut-sized balls.

Place a steamer basket in the bottom of a large pan. Add water to just below the bottom of the steamer basket. Bring water to a boil. Place

Italian Meatball Sub
(*continued*)

meatballs in basket leaving ½-inch between meatballs, cooking in batches if needed. Cover pan with tight-fitting lid and steam meatballs until done, about 15 minutes.

Place cooked meatballs in a colander to drain.

Assembling Subs:

In a large frying pan, sauté the meatballs with ¼ cup of oil until browned.

Add Marinara Sauce.

Place oven rack in center position and turn on oven broiler to high.

Place sub rolls in a large baking dish with cut edge facing up.

Fill sub rolls with meatballs and sauce. Top with cheese.

Place baking dish on middle rack and broil subs until cheese is melted, about two minutes.

Jambalaya

This famous New Orleans Fat Tuesday entrée is a blend of French, Spanish, and African cuisines.

Yield: 5 servings

4 cups cooked Brown Rice (pg. 85)

1 red bell pepper, medium dice

1 small sweet onion, medium dice

¼ cup vegetable oil

14 oz. vegan kielbasa sausage, large dice

2 Tbs. Cajun Seasoning (pg. 140)

15-oz. can black-eyed peas, drained and rinsed

14-oz. can crushed tomatoes

¼ cup water

Salt to taste (about 1 tsp.)

Prepare rice and set aside.

In a large pan, sauté the bell pepper and onion with the oil until tender.

Add sausage and Cajun Seasoning and cook for one minute.

Add black-eyed peas, crushed tomatoes, and water.

Bring to a low boil and simmer for 10 minutes.

Add salt to taste.

Combine with rice or serve over rice.

Jamaica

Jerk Tofu

This Caribbean dish can be served with Jamaican Rice and Peas (pg. 92) and/or Cornmeal Coo Coo (pg. 88).

Yield: 4 servings

Juice of 2 oranges (1 cup)

Juice of 1 lime (2 Tbs.)

¼ cup soy sauce

3 green onions, chopped

1 tomato, medium dice

16 oz. extra firm tofu

2 Tbs. Jerk Seasoning*

Preheat oven to 325°F.

In a small bowl, combine orange juice, lime juice, soy sauce, green onions, and tomato. Set aside.

Cut tofu into four slabs.

Rub jerk seasoning on all sides of tofu.

Place tofu in a 9-inch × 13-inch baking dish.

Pour orange juice mixture over tofu.

Bake for 45 minutes.

***Jerk Seasoning**

Yield: 2 Tbs.

1 tsp. allspice

1 tsp. thyme

½ tsp. garlic powder

½ tsp. black pepper

½ tsp. cinnamon

½ tsp. salt

¼ tsp. cayenne

In a small bowl, combine all ingredients.

Kung Pao Eggplant

This classic Sichuan dish is named after Ding Baozhen (1820-1886) of the Qing Dynasty (1644–1911).

Yield: 6 servings

2 cups Kung Pao Sauce (pg. 302)

2 eggplants

1¼ cups flour

¼ cup cornstarch

1 Tbs. salt

1½ tsp. egg replacer powder

1½ tsp. baking powder

1¼ cups soy milk

Vegetable oil for frying

½ cup chopped green onions

½ cup chopped peanuts

Prepare Kung Pao Sauce and keep warm until needed.

Peel eggplant, cut into ½-inch rounds, and set aside.

In a large shallow bowl, combine flour, cornstarch, salt, egg replacer powder, and baking powder. Whisk in soy milk.

Add ¼-inch of oil to a large skillet.

Heat oil to 350°F.

Lightly batter eggplant and place in hot oil (cooking in batches if needed).

Cook eggplant until golden brown on each side.

Serve eggplant topped with Kung Pao Sauce, green onions, and peanuts.

Serve with Brown Rice (pg. 85) or Jasmine Rice (pg. 93).

Lasagna

Yield: 8 servings

12 lasagna noodles

1 onion, small dice

¼ cup olive oil

2 Tbs. basil

1 Tbs. onion powder

1 Tbs. garlic powder

1 Tbs. oregano

1 Tbs. salt

1 tsp. sugar

14 oz. soy ground

28-oz. can crushed tomatoes

12 oz. tomato paste

1 cup water

20 oz. vegan mozzarella, shredded

Preheat oven to 325°F.

Boil lasagna noodles just until soft, about six minutes. Do not overcook noodles (slightly undercooked is ideal). Drain off water and place cooked noodles in cold water until ready to be used.

In a large saucepan, sauté the onion with the oil until tender.

Add basil, onion powder, garlic powder, oregano, salt, sugar, and soy ground. Cook until soy ground is broken up and hot.

Add crushed tomatoes, tomato paste and water. Cook until hot.

Drain cold water from noodles.

Spread one cup of sauce on the bottom of a 9-inch × 13-inch baking dish.

Layer dish with four noodles, two cups of sauce, and 1¼ cups of cheese.

Repeat two more times.

Bake, covered, for 55 minutes.

Uncover and let cool for 20 minutes before serving.

Mushroom Leek Galette

Yield: Two 9-inch galettes (6 servings)

Filling:

6 cups sliced mushrooms (1 lb.)

4 cups chopped leeks (2 leeks)

1½ cups chopped shallots

¼ cup olive oil

1 tsp. thyme

1 tsp. garlic powder

½ tsp. black pepper

¼ cup flour

½ cup vegan sour cream

Salt to taste (about 1 tsp.)

Pastry:

1½ cups flour

½ tsp. salt

½ cup vegan sour cream

¼ cup olive oil

Waxed paper

Filling:

In a large saucepan, sauté the mushrooms, leeks, and shallots with the oil until most of the mushroom liquid has evaporated (about 20 minutes).

Add thyme, garlic powder, black pepper, and flour. Cook for one minute.

Add ½ cup sour cream.

Add salt to taste.

Chill filling.

Pastry:

In a large bowl, mix the flour and salt.

Mushroom Leek Galette
(*continued*)

Stir in the sour cream and oil just until combined.

Divided dough into two balls.

Assemble Galette:

Between two pieces of waxed paper, roll each dough ball into a 12-inch circle.

Remove waxed paper and place dough on a baking sheet.

Place half of the filling in the center of each dough circle, leaving 1½-inches of bare dough around the edge.

Gather the edge of each galette up and over the edge of the filling, creating an open-faced galette.

Preheat oven to 425°F.

Bake for 25 minutes.

Mushroom Stroganoff

This dish is named after Russian diplomat Count Paul Stroganov, who reached the rank of Lieutenant General and commanded an army during the Napoleonic campaigns of 1811–1815.

Yield: 6 servings

1 onion, small dice

½ cup vegetable oil

7 cups large diced mushrooms (1½ lbs.)

½ tsp. thyme

½ tsp. onion powder

⅛ tsp. black pepper

⅛ tsp. nutmeg

¾ cup flour

4 cups mushroom broth

1½ cups vegan sour cream, divided

Salt to taste (about 1½ tsp.)

12 oz. uncooked rotelle pasta

In a large pan, sauté the onion with the oil until tender.

Add mushrooms, thyme, onion powder, black pepper, and nutmeg.

Cook until mushrooms have softened.

Add flour and cook one minute.

Add broth.

Heat until thickened, stirring constantly.

Stir in one cup of the sour cream.

Add salt to taste.

Cook pasta according to package directions.

Serve sauce over pasta and garnish with remaining sour cream.

Ireland

O'Brian's Biscuit Stew

Yield: 8 servings

2 medium russet potatoes, peeled and medium dice

¼ cup vegetable oil

1 carrot, medium dice

3 stalks celery, medium dice

1 onion, small dice

⅓ cup flour

1 tsp. onion powder

½ tsp. thyme

15-oz. can white kidney or navy beans, drained and rinsed

4 cups vegetable broth

Salt to taste (about 2 tsp.)

Black pepper to taste (about ¼ tsp.)

Drop Biscuit Dough (pg. 327)

Boil potatoes just until soft. Drain off water and set aside.

In a large saucepan, sauté the carrot, celery, and onion with the oil until tender.

Add flour, onion powder, and thyme. Sauté for two minutes.

Add beans, potatoes, and vegetable broth.

Bring stew to a boil, reduce heat to low, and simmer for 10 minutes, stirring frequently.

Add salt and pepper to taste.

Preheat oven to 400°F.

While stew is simmering, prepare Biscuit Dough.

Pour stew into a 10-inch × 15-inch baking dish.

Drop 15 scoops of biscuit dough on top of the stew and slightly push into the stew.

Bake for 20 minutes, or until a toothpick inserted in the middle of a biscuit comes out clean.

Orange Tofu

This spicy dish originated in Hunan. The American version of this dish is sweeter and the tofu is fried.

Yield: 4 servings

4 cups cooked Brown Rice (pg. 85)

2 cups prepared Spicy Orange Sauce (pg. 313)

16 oz. extra firm tofu, large dice

¼ cup cornstarch

½ tsp. salt

¼ cup vegetable oil

1 bunch green onions, chopped

Prepare rice and set aside.

Prepare Spicy Orange Sauce and set aside.

Toss tofu with cornstarch and salt.

In a large pan, sauté the tofu with the oil until crisp on all sides.

Stir in orange sauce.

Serve over rice.

Garnish with green onions.

Pad Thai

Yield: 3 servings

2½ cups Pad Thai Sauce, divided (pg. 306)

8 oz. rice noodles

14 oz. extra firm tofu, medium dice

2 Tbs. vegetable oil

1 bunch green onions, chopped

8 oz. bean sprouts, thoroughly rinsed

⅓ cup chopped peanuts

1 whole lime, wedged

Vegan sriracha sauce

Additional garnish options: matchstick or shredded carrots, chopped cashews or almonds, shredded red or green cabbage, chopped Thai basil, chopped sweet basil, chopped cilantro, roasted garlic, shelled edamame, raw or roasted sliced red onions, roasted or fresh chopped jalapeños or other hot peppers

Prepare Pad Thai Sauce and set aside.

Soak rice noodles in hot tap water until soft, about 10-30 minutes. Drain off water and set aside.

In a large pan, lightly fry tofu with oil.

Add rice noodles and 1½ cups of the Pad Thai Sauce.

Cook until sauce has been absorbed into the noodles and noodles are tender, about seven minutes. Add additional Pad Thai Sauce as needed.

Add green onions and bean sprouts.

Cook until hot.

Place in a large serving dish and garnish.

Papa Rellenos

This is a mashed-potato-wrapped version of Chili Rellenos. The recipe is a bit time consuming, but so worth it!

Yield: 12-14 rellenos

2 cups Enchilada Sauce (pg. 299)

1¼ cups vegan Ricotta Cheese (pg. 335)

3 7-oz. cans whole green chilies, drained

4 3½-inch russet potatoes, peeled and quartered (about 1½ pounds before peeling)

2 tsp. salt

Flour for working into dough, about 1-2 cups

Vegetable oil for frying

Prepare Enchilada Sauce and set aside.

Prepare Ricotta Cheese and set aside.

Remove any blackened bits from chilies and discard the bits.

Fill chilies with Ricotta Cheese (using a pastry bag makes this easier) and set aside on two layers of paper towels.

Place potatoes in a large saucepan, cover with water, and boil until tender.

Drain off water. Mash potatoes with salt until smooth.

Stir in enough flour so potatoes are no longer sticky and have a playdough-like consistency.

Count number of chilies on hand. Divide potato dough into the same number of chilies on hand. Place dough balls on a well-floured surface.

On the well-floured surface, roll one piece of dough into a 6-inch × 4-inch piece.

Wrap one cheese-stuffed-chili with potato dough, completely covering chili. Place on a well-floured surface.

Repeat with remaining chilies and dough.

Papa Rellenos
(*continued*)

Add ¼-inch of oil to a large skillet.

Heat oil to 350°F.

Cook rellenos until golden brown on each side.

Top with Enchilada Sauce just before serving.

Pasta Alexander

Yield: 5 servings

1 medium sweet onion, small dice

¼ cup olive oil

1 tsp. basil

1 tsp. onion powder

½ tsp. oregano

¼ tsp. black pepper

¼ cup balsamic vinegar

8 sun-dried tomatoes, julienne cut

15-oz. can diced tomatoes

8 oz. frozen artichoke hearts, thawed and medium dice

15-oz. can cannellini beans, drained and rinsed

2 cups vegetable broth

Salt to taste (about 2 tsp.)

14 oz. bow tie pasta (farfalle) or Homemade Pasta (pg. 331)

In a large pan, sauté the onion with the oil until tender.

Add basil, onion powder, oregano, and black pepper.

Add vinegar and cook until vinegar is reduced by half.

Add sun-dried tomatoes, canned tomatoes, artichoke hearts, beans, and vegetable broth. Bring to a boil. Simmer until sun-dried tomatoes are soft.

Add salt to taste and keep warm.

Cook pasta according to package directions.

Toss pasta with sauce.

Pasta Bolognese

Yield: 6 servings

½ onion, small dice

1 carrot, small dice

2 stalks celery, small dice

¼ cup olive oil

1 Tbs. basil

2 tsp. onion powder

2 tsp. oregano

1 tsp. sugar

¼ cup balsamic vinegar

1 cup vegetable broth

6 oz. soy ground

28-oz. can crushed tomatoes

Salt to taste (about 1 tsp.)

14 oz. uncooked pasta

In a 3-quart saucepan, sauté the onion, carrot, and celery with the olive oil until tender.

Add the basil, onion powder, oregano, and sugar and sauté for one minute.

Add balsamic vinegar and cook for two minutes, stirring often.

Add vegetable broth and cook until vegetable broth is reduced by half, about five minutes.

Add soy ground and crushed tomatoes.

Heat until hot, stirring often.

Reduce heat to low and simmer for 10 minutes, stirring occasionally.

Add salt to taste.

Cook pasta according to package directions. Serve sauce over pasta.

Pesto Pasta

Yield: 4 servings

15 peeled cloves of garlic (one whole garlic bulb)

½ cup olive oil

¼ cup pine nuts or walnuts

¾ tsp. salt

2 bunches basil, stemmed

12 oz. uncooked penne pasta

Preheat oven to 375°F.

In a small baking dish, toss garlic with olive oil.

Bake for 20 minutes.

Cool garlic and roasting oil in the refrigerator for 30 minutes.

In a food processor, combine roasted garlic with its roasting oil, pine nuts or walnuts, and salt until smooth.

Add basil and pulse blade just until smooth.

Cook pasta according to package directions.

Drain and then toss pasta with Pesto Sauce.

Place in a sauté pan and heat just until hot.

Mayan

Plantains with Mole Sauce

The Mayans are believed to have discovered and cultivated cacao (chocolate), which is in the mole sauce.

Yield: 4 servings

4 servings Polenta, firm style (pg. 95)

2 cups Mole Sauce (pg. 305)

2 yellow plantains

Vegetable oil for grilling

2 cups cold salt water (2 cups water and 2 Tbs. salt)

2 tsp. seasoned salt (1½ tsp. garlic powder or onion powder and ½ tsp. salt)

15-oz. can black beans, drained and rinsed

Salt to taste

Prepare Polenta. Keep warm in a preheated 170°F oven.

Prepare Mole Sauce. Keep warm in the preheated 170°F oven.

Peel plantains and slice diagonally into ½-inch thick slices.

Preheat oil in large skillet. Grill plantains with oil until browned, about two minutes on each side (save oil for step eight).

Place fried plantains in salt water mixture for one minute.

Remove plantains and pat dry with paper towels.

On a cutting board and using the palm of your hand, slightly squash plantains to almost half as thick.

In a large skillet, re-grill plantains with oil for an additional two minutes on each side.

Remove from skillet and toss with seasoned salt.

In a 2-quart saucepan, heat black beans. Add salt if needed.

To serve, place polenta on plate and top with black beans, grilled plantains, and Mole Sauce.

Portobello Mushroom Wellington

The inspiration for this dish came from national hero Arthur Wellesley who defeated Napoleon at Waterloo in 1815 and went on to become the first Duke of Wellington. Serve with Dijon Sauce (pg. 297) if desired.

Yield: 4 servings

½ onion, small dice

2 Tbs. olive oil

2 Tbs. minced garlic

1 bunch spinach, chopped

½ tsp. salt

4 portobello mushrooms, stemmed

1 9-inch X 9-inch vegan puff pastry sheet, thawed

Olive oil for brushing

Sauté the onion with the two Tbs. olive oil until tender.

Add garlic and sauté until tender.

Add spinach and salt and cook until spinach is wilted.

Divide spinach mixture into four portions and chill in refrigerator.

Preheat oven to 450°F.

Brush tops of mushrooms with olive oil.

Place mushrooms in a baking dish with underside of mushrooms facing down.

Bake mushrooms until soft, about 10-15 minutes.

Pat mushrooms dry, lightly squeezing if needed.

Chill mushrooms.

Cut puff pastry into four equal squares.

Place one puff pastry square on counter.

Place one mushroom with underside facing up on the puff pastry square.

Place one portion of spinach mixture on mushroom.

Portobello Mushroom Wellington
(*continued*)

Pull edges of pastry around mushroom and spinach mixture until they touch.

Turn right side up (so gathered edge is touching baking dish) and place on an oiled baking dish.

Brush top of puff pastry with olive oil.

Repeat with remaining pastry, mushrooms, and spinach.

Bake at 450°F until browned, about 15-20 minutes.

Puttanesca

Yield: 3 servings

14-oz. can quartered artichoke hearts, drained and medium dice

6-oz. can sliced black olives, drained

6 cups medium diced fresh tomatoes

1 onion, small dice

6 cloves garlic, peeled, crushed, and minced

¼ cup olive oil

¼ cup balsamic vinegar

1 tsp. basil

1 tsp. oregano

¼ tsp. black pepper

¼ tsp. red pepper flakes

Salt to taste (about 1½ tsp.)

8 oz. uncooked penne pasta

¼ cup chopped fresh basil (optional)

Preheat oven to 475°F.

In a large bowl, combine artichoke hearts, olives, tomatoes, onion, garlic, olive oil, balsamic vinegar, basil, oregano, black pepper, and red pepper flakes.

Divide between two 10-inch × 15-inch baking dishes.

Bake for 35 minutes. Stirring every 10 minutes.

Remove veggies from oven and place in a large mixing bowl.

Add salt to taste.

Reduce oven temperature to 170°F.

Puttanesca
(*continued*)

Return veggies to a single baking dish and place in oven to keep warm.

Cook pasta according to package instructions.

Combine veggies with pasta.

Top with chopped basil.

Quiche Lorraine

Dating back to the mid 1500s, Quiche Lorraine was a recipe handed down from mother to daughter in the Lorraine region of France.

Yield: One 9-inch pie

1 9-inch single precooked Pie Crust (pg. 334)

16 oz. extra firm tofu

1 onion, small dice

2 Tbs. vegetable oil

7 oz. tempeh bacon*, small dice

12 oz. vegan cheese (Swiss, jack, or mozzarella), shredded

1 tsp. salt

⅛ tsp. cayenne pepper

** Substitute with ¾ cup chopped Seitan Bacon (pg. 127) if preferred.*

Preheat oven to 350°F.

Prepare pie crust and set aside.

In a food processor, process tofu until smooth. Transfer to a large bowl and set aside.

In a 3-quart saucepan, sauté the onion with the oil until tender.

Add tempeh and sauté one minute.

Add sautéed onions and tempeh to the tofu.

Add shredded cheese, salt and cayenne pepper.

Spoon mixture into pie crust.

Bake for 45 minutes.

Reuben Sandwich

Yield: 4 sandwiches

Corned Beef (pg. 151)

½ cup vegan Thousand Island Dressing (pg. 80)

1 cup well-drained sauerkraut

8 slices vegan rye bread

4 slices vegan Swiss or jack cheese

¼ cup softened vegan margarine

Prepare Corned Beef and then slice off 12 thin slices to make sandwiches.

Prepare Thousand Island Dressing and set aside.

Preheat electric griddle or skillet to 350°F, or put on medium-low heat if using a stovetop griddle or skillet.

Grill corned beef slices with sauerkraut until warm.

Place corned beef and sauerkraut on four slices of bread. Top with Thousand Island dressing and cheese.

Place remaining bread on top.

Spread margarine on outside of each slice of bread.

Grill sandwiches until browned on each side.

If cheese is not melted, place sandwiches briefly in microwave or place open-faced under broiler.

Roasted Vegetable Pizza with Pesto Sauce

Yield: One 14-inch pizza

Pizza Dough (slow, or fast-rise method (pg. 239 or pg. 238)

½ cup Pesto Sauce (pg. 308)

1 cup medium diced onions

1 cup medium diced red bell peppers

1 cup halved white mushrooms

1 cup medium diced zucchini

½ tsp. salt

1 Tbs. olive oil

Pan spray

Prepare Pizza Dough and set aside.

Prepare Pesto Sauce and set aside.

Roll dough into a 14-inch round.

Place on a pan-sprayed baking sheet. Cover and set aside.

Preheat oven to 450°F.

In a large bowl, combine onions, bell peppers, mushrooms, zucchini, salt, and olive oil.

Place in a baking dish and bake until lightly browned on the edges, about 20 minutes.

Spread Pesto Sauce on pizza dough.

Add roasted vegetables.

Bake pizza at 450°F until dough is cooked, about 15 minutes.

Roasted Yam Enchiladas with Tomatillo Sauce

Tomatillos are often referred to as Mexican tomatoes. Fresh tomatillos have a parchment-like husk which needs to be removed before using.

Yield: 12 enchiladas

2 cups Tomatillo Sauce (pg. 320)

4 cups medium diced peeled yams

1 medium sweet onion, small dice

2 Tbs. vegetable oil

1 tsp. salt

12 6-inch Corn Tortillas (pg. 230)

Vegetable oil for brushing

Prepare Tomatillo Sauce and set aside.

Preheat oven to 450°F.

In a baking dish, combine yams, onion, 2 Tbs. vegetable oil, and salt.

Bake for 30 minutes, stirring every 10 minutes. Set aside.

Soften tortillas by brushing each tortilla with vegetable oil and placing on a warm griddle or in a microwave just until softened.

Place ¼ cup of roasted yam mixture in the middle of each tortilla.

Roll up and place in a large baking dish, seam side down.

Cover enchiladas with Tomatillo Sauce.

Bake until hot, about 10 minutes.

Sicilian Style Pizza

Sicilian pizza has a thick soft crust, is cooked in a square or rectangular pan, has just a few ingredients, and usually includes fresh herbs.

Yield: 6 servings

1 batch fast-rise Pizza Dough (pg. 238)

½ cup Pizza Sauce (pg. 310)

1 sweet onion, small dice

1 Tbs. olive oil

4 oz. vegan pepperoni

10 oz. vegan mozzarella, shredded

¼ cup chopped fresh basil

Prepare Pizza Dough and set aside.

Prepare Pizza Sauce and set aside.

Sauté the onion with the oil until tender. Set aside.

Roll out pizza dough to 11-inches × 15-inches.

Press dough into an oiled 9-inch × 13-inch baking dish with 1 inch of dough going up the edges.

Spread Pizza Sauce on dough including edges.

Add pepperoni, onion, cheese, and basil.

Cover and let rise for 30 minutes.

Preheat oven to 450°F.

Bake until crust is cooked, about 15 minutes.

If cheese is not fully melted, set oven broiler on high and broil until cheese is melted, about two minutes. Do not walk away from oven while cheese is broiling because it can burn quickly.

Spare Ribz with Plum Sauce

Yield: 4 servings

4 cups cooked Brown Rice (pg. 85)

2 cups prepared Plum Sauce, divided (pg. 311)

1⅓ cups vital wheat gluten flour

1 Tbs. paprika

1 tsp. ginger powder

1 tsp. onion powder

1¼ tsp. salt

1 cup water

6 Tbs. vegetable oil, divided

2 Tbs. soy sauce

1 tsp. liquid smoke

½ onion, thin julienne cut

1 red bell pepper, thin julienne cut

12 snow peas, thin julienne cut

Pan spray

Prepare rice and set aside.

Prepare Plum Sauce and set aside.

Preheat oven to 325°F.

In a large bowl, whisk together the vital wheat gluten flour, paprika, ginger, onion powder, and salt.

Add water, three Tbs. oil, soy sauce, and liquid smoke. Stir just until combined.

Press dough into a pan-sprayed 8-inch × 8-inch baking dish.

Bake for 40 minutes.

Remove seitan from baking dish and cut into ¼-inch × 3-inch strips.

Place strips, onion, bell pepper, and snow peas in a

large frying pan and sauté with remaining three Tbs. of oil until crisp.

Add 1¼ cups of the Plum Sauce.

Served over rice with remaining Plum Sauce on the side.

USA

State Fair Corn Dogs

Texan Neil Fletcher created the corn dog at the 1942 state fair. Serve with ketchup and mustard.

Yield: 10 baked* or fried corn dogs**

10 6-inch bamboo skewers

10 vegan hot dogs

1¾ cups soy milk

2¾ tsp. salt

1 Tbs. vegetable oil

1½ cups cornmeal

1 cup flour

1 Tbs. baking powder

Vegetable oil for frying

Insert skewers lengthwise and half way into hot dogs and set aside.

In a 3-quart saucepan, combine soy milk, salt, and oil and bring to a boil.

Slowly whisk in cornmeal. Stirring constantly, cook on low until thickened, about one minute.

Remove from heat, cover, and let sit for 10 minutes.

Transfer to a mixing bowl.

Stir in flour and baking powder.

Divided dough into 10 pieces.

On a lightly floured surface, press out a piece of dough to make a 4-inch × 5-inch piece. Place one hot dog in the middle of the dough and form dough around hot dog. Roll until edges are smooth.

Choose either the baked or fried method below:

**Baked method:*
Preheat oven to 425°F. Place Corn Dogs on an oiled baking dish. Brush with oil. Bake for 17 minutes.

***Fried method:*
Preheat ¼-inch of oil in a skillet or recommended amount of oil in a deep fat fryer to 350°F. Fry Corn Dogs until golden brown on each side, turning as necessary.

Stromboli

Stromboli got its name from the 1950 movie Stromboli. *Romano's Pizza Shop of Essington, PA, created the dish.*

Yield: 6

Pizza Dough, slow-rise (pg. 239)

1 cup Pizza Sauce (pg. 310)

1¼ cups vegan Ricotta Cheese (pg. 335)

1 onion, small dice

2 Tbs. olive oil

2 oz. vegan pepperoni

Olive oil for brushing

Prepare Pizza Dough and set aside.

Prepare Pizza Sauce and set aside.

Prepare Ricotta Cheese and set aside.

In a small saucepan, sauté the onion with the oil until tender.

In a bowl, combine sautéed onion, pepperoni, Pizza Sauce, and Ricotta Cheese. Set aside.

On a lightly floured surface, roll pizza dough into a 12-inch × 18-inch rectangle.

Spread the mixture evenly on the dough up to ½-inch of the edge.

Roll-up dough into an 18-inch log.

Connect ends of log together and place on an oiled baking sheet.

Brush with olive oil.

Preheat oven to 375°F.

Bake until dough is cooked, about 35 minutes.

Brush with additional olive oil.

Sun-dried Tomato Pasta

Sun-dried tomatoes, also known as love apples, were at one time dried on tile roofs in Italy to preserve them for winter use.

Yield: 5 servings

12 sun-dried tomatoes (not the ones packed in oil)

½ onion, small dice

⅓ cup olive oil

1 Tbs. basil

2 tsp. oregano

1 tsp. garlic powder

1 tsp. onion powder

1 tsp. sugar

⅛ tsp. black pepper

½ cup flour

¼ cup nutritional yeast flakes

4 cups unsweetened soy milk

Salt to taste (about 2 tsp.)

16 oz. uncooked penne pasta

10 oz. vegan mozzarella, shredded

Boil sun-dried tomatoes for eight minutes and drain off water.

Small dice the tomatoes and set aside.

In a 3-quart saucepan, sauté the onion with the oil until tender.

Add basil, oregano, garlic powder, onion powder, sugar, black pepper, and flour. Cook for one minute.

Stir in nutritional yeast flakes and sun-dried tomatoes.

Stir in soy milk.

Cook sauce until hot and thickened, stirring constantly.

Add salt to taste and set aside.

Sun-dried Tomato Pasta
(*continued*)

Cook pasta according to package directions.

Combine sauce with pasta.

Pour into an 8-inch × 10-inch baking dish.

Top with shredded cheese.

Preheat oven broiler setting to high.

Place baking dish on middle rack.

Broil until cheese is melted, about two minutes. Do not walk away from oven while cheese is broiling because it can burn quickly.

Swedish Meatballs

This dish is often served on smorgasbords with traditional sour cream sauce and lingonberry preserves. These meatballs can be served alone or with pasta, mashed potatoes, or rice.

Yield: 4 servings

24 Meatballs (pg. 329) or 16 oz. vegan meatballs

½ onion, small dice

¼ cup vegetable oil

1 tsp. onion powder

½ tsp. thyme

¼ tsp. black pepper

¼ tsp. nutmeg

⅓ cup flour

2 cups vegetable broth

12 oz. vegan sour cream

Salt to taste (about ¾ tsp.)

Prepare Meatballs or heat packaged meatballs according to directions. Set aside.

In a large pan, sauté the onion with the oil until tender.

Add onion powder, thyme, black pepper, nutmeg, and flour.

Add vegetable broth.

Cook until hot and thickened, stirring frequently.

Add sour cream and cook until hot.

Add meatballs and cook until hot.

Add salt to taste.

Sweet and Sour Ribz

Yield: 4 servings

4 cups cooked Brown Rice (pg. 85)

2 cups Sweet and Sour Sauce (pg. 314)

1¼ cups vital wheat gluten flour

1 Tbs. paprika

1 tsp. ginger powder

1 tsp. onion powder

1 tsp. salt

1 cup water

6 Tbs. vegetable oil, divided

Pan spray

Prepare rice and set aside.

Prepare Sweet and Sour Sauce and set aside.

Preheat oven to 325°F.

In a large bowl, whisk together the vital wheat gluten flour, paprika, ginger powder, onion powder, and salt.

Add water and three Tbs. of the oil. Mix just until combined.

Press into a pan-sprayed 8-inch × 8-inch baking dish.

Bake for 40 minutes.

Remove seitan from baking dish and cut into ¼-inch × 3-inch strips.

Place strips in a large frying pan and sauté with remaining three Tbs. of oil until crispy.

Add sweet and sour sauce.

Serve over rice.

Tamales

A sweet version filled with fruit is also made in Mexico as a dessert.

Yield: 20 tamales

20 dried corn husks

3 cups masa flour

2¾ tsp. salt, divided

2¼ cups vegetable broth

⅓ cup vegetable oil

3 Tbs. vegetable oil

1 large sweet onion, small dice

15-oz. can black beans, drained and rinsed

15-oz. can hominy, drained and rinsed

1 tsp. onion powder

Optional sauces:
Enchilada Sauce (pg. 299), Ancho Sauce (pg. 285), Mole Sauce (pg. 305), or Tomatillo Sauce (pg. 320)

Optional toppings:
sour cream, Guacamole (pg. 300), salsa

Soak husks in warm water until soft, about 20 minutes. Drain, rinse, and set aside.

In a large bowl, combine masa, 1¾ tsp. of the salt, vegetable broth, and ⅓ cup oil. Set aside.

In a 3-quart saucepan, sauté the onion with the three Tbs. of oil until tender. Add black beans, hominy, onion powder, and the remaining one tsp. of salt. Set aside.

Spread three Tbs. of the masa mixture on the large bottom half of a corn husk.

Add three Tbs. of the black bean mixture in the middle of the masa layer.

Roll up corn husk lengthwise.

Fold over the top of the corn husk and place on a baking sheet.

Repeat with remaining husks, masa, and black bean filling.

Tamales
(*continued*)

In a steamer basket, lay down the tamales so they crisscross each other, leaving room for the steam to circulate around them.

Cover with a tight-fitting lid and steam for two hours or until filling is set.

Prepare sauce if preferred.

Remove tamales from steamer and let cool for 10 minutes.

Remove husks.

Serve with sauce and/or choice of toppings.

Tandoori Tofu

Serve with Pita (pg. 237) or Naan (pg. 236), and/or Raita (pg. 312) if preferred.

Yield: 4 servings

4 cups cooked Brown Rice (pg. 85)

16 oz. extra firm tofu, cut into 4 slabs

1 cup plain soy yogurt

1 Tbs. curry powder

1 tsp. paprika

½ tsp. salt

¼ tsp. cayenne pepper

Preheat oven to 400°F.

Prepare rice and set aside.

In a small bowl, combine yogurt, curry powder, paprika, salt, and cayenne pepper.

Place tofu in a 9-inch × 13-inch baking dish.

Spread yogurt mixture over tofu.

Bake for 30 minutes.

Serve over rice.

Thai Lentils with Sweet Potatoes

Thai basil is quickly identified by its purple stems and subtle licorice-mint flavor.

Yield: 6 servings

4 cups cooked Brown Rice (pg. 85)

1 small sweet potato, peeled and small dice

½ onion, small dice

1 red bell pepper, small dice

3 Tbs. olive oil

1 Tbs. fresh minced ginger

2 Tbs. vegan yellow or red curry paste

1½ cups uncooked lentils, rinsed

4 cups water

2 tomatoes, medium dice

Salt to taste (about 1¼ tsp.)

Juice of one lime

1 bunch Thai basil*, stems removed and leaves lightly chopped

** Use sweet basil or cilantro if you prefer.*

Prepare rice and set aside.

In a 3-quart saucepan, sauté the sweet potato, onion, and pepper with the oil until tender.

Add ginger and cook until tender, about two minutes.

Add curry paste and cook for one minute.

Add lentils, water, and tomatoes.

Bring to a boil and reduce heat to low. Cover and simmer until lentils are tender, (about one hour) stirring occasionally.

Add salt to taste.

Add lime juice.

Serve over rice.

Garnish with basil.

Thai Tempeh with Jasmine Rice

Spicy chilies were introduced to Thailand by Portuguese missionaries in the late 1600s.

Yield: 3 servings

4 cups cooked Jasmine Rice (pg. 93)

2 cups Thai Coconut Sauce (pg. 318)

½ cup flour

1 tsp. paprika

1 tsp. onion powder

1 tsp. salt

½ cup soy milk

8 oz. tempeh, cut into 6 pieces

Vegetable oil for grilling

Prepare rice and set aside.

Prepare Thai Coconut Sauce and set aside.

On a dinner plate, combine flour, paprika, onion powder, and salt.

On a second dinner plate, add soy milk.

Dredge tempeh in soy milk and then in the flour mixture.

On a hot oiled griddle, grill tempeh until browned on each side.

Serve grilled tempeh on top of rice with Thai Coconut Sauce.

Thai Tofu with Coconut Sauce

Yield: 4 servings

4 cups cooked Brown Rice (pg. 85)

2 cups Thai Coconut Sauce (pg. 318)

⅓ cup cornstarch

1 tsp. paprika

1 tsp. onion powder

1 tsp. salt

16 oz. extra firm tofu, large dice

¼ cup vegetable oil

1 red bell pepper, thin julienne cut

1 medium sweet onion, thin julienne cut

2 cups sliced broccoli

1 bunch Thai or sweet basil stemmed and thin julienne cut

Prepare rice and set aside.

Prepare Thai Coconut Sauce and set aside.

In a bowl, combine cornstarch, paprika, onion powder, and salt.

Coat tofu with cornstarch mixture.

In a large pan, sauté the tofu with the oil until crisp on all sides (save oil for next step). Set aside.

Sauté red bell pepper, sweet onion, and broccoli until tender. Add additional oil if needed.

Add tofu and heat until hot.

Add coconut sauce and heat until hot.

Serve on top of rice.

Garnish with basil.

Thai Tortilla Wrap

Yield: 8 wraps

2 cups cooked Brown Rice (pg. 85)

1½ cups Coconut Peanut Sauce (pg. 294)

8 oz. ready-to-eat teriyaki tofu

1 cup shredded purple cabbage

1 cup shredded carrot

1 bunch Thai or sweet basil, stemmed and chopped

8 8-inch Flour Tortillas (pg. 234)

Prepare rice and set aside.

Prepare Coconut Peanut Sauce and set aside.

Cut tofu into 16 strips and set aside.

In a bowl, combine cabbage, carrot, and basil.

Soften tortillas in microwave or on a hot griddle.

Fill each tortilla with ¼ cup rice, three Tbs. sauce, and ½ cup vegetable mixture.

Roll burrito style.

Vegetable Pot Pie

In 1951 the company Swanson made the frozen pot pie available for retail sale.

Yield: 6 servings

1 single Pie Crust* (pg. 334)

3 small russet potatoes, peeled and medium dice

2 carrots, medium dice

3 celery stalks, medium dice

½ onion, small dice

⅓ cup vegetable oil

1 tsp. onion powder

½ tsp. thyme

¼ tsp. black pepper

½ cup flour

15-oz. can kidney beans, drained and rinsed

1¾ cups vegetable broth

Salt to taste (about 1½ tsp.)

** If you prefer a bottom and top crust to the pot pie, use the double Pie Crust recipe (pg. 332).*

Prepare pie crust. Line a 9-inch pie dish with pie crust. Cover and set aside.

Boil potatoes just until soft, about 12 minutes. Drain off water and set potatoes aside.

In a large pan, sauté the carrots, celery, and onion with the oil until tender.

Add onion powder, thyme, pepper, and flour.

Add potatoes, beans, and vegetable broth and heat until thickened, stirring frequently.

Add salt to taste.

Preheat oven to 425°F.

Add stew to pie crust and add top crust if making a two crust pie.

Bake for 30 minutes.

Portugal

Vegetable Vindaloo

Although a popular dish in India, vindaloo originated in Portugal and was brought to India by sailors. In Portuguese "alho" refers to garlic, and in Hindi "aloo" means potato, hence the confusion on whether or not to add potatoes. Serve with Pita (pg. 237) or Naan (pg. 236) if preferred.

Yield: 5 servings

4 cups cooked Brown Rice (pg. 85)

3 cups medium diced yellow potatoes

1 small red onion, small dice

¼ cup olive oil

4 cloves garlic, peeled, crushed, and minced

2 tsp. cayenne pepper or to taste

1 tsp. paprika

1 tsp. cumin

1 tsp. garam masala

½ tsp. turmeric

½ tsp. onion powder

½ tsp. garlic powder

¼ tsp. ground cardamom

¼ cup water

15-oz. can garbanzo beans, drained and rinsed

15-oz. can diced tomatoes

2 Tbs. wine vinegar

2 Tbs. tamarind paste

Salt to taste (about 1½ tsp.)

Garnish options:
diced red onions, chopped cilantro, chopped jalapeño, lime wedges, Raita (pg. 312)

Prepare rice and set aside.

Boil potatoes just until tender, about 15 minutes. Drain and set aside.

Vegetable Vindaloo
(*continued*)

In a large pan, sauté the onion with the oil until tender.

Add garlic and sauté for two minutes.

Add herbs and sauté for one minute.

Add water, garbanzo beans, tomatoes, vinegar, tamarind paste, and potatoes.

Simmer for 10 minutes.

Add salt to taste.

Served over rice.

Garnish if preferred.

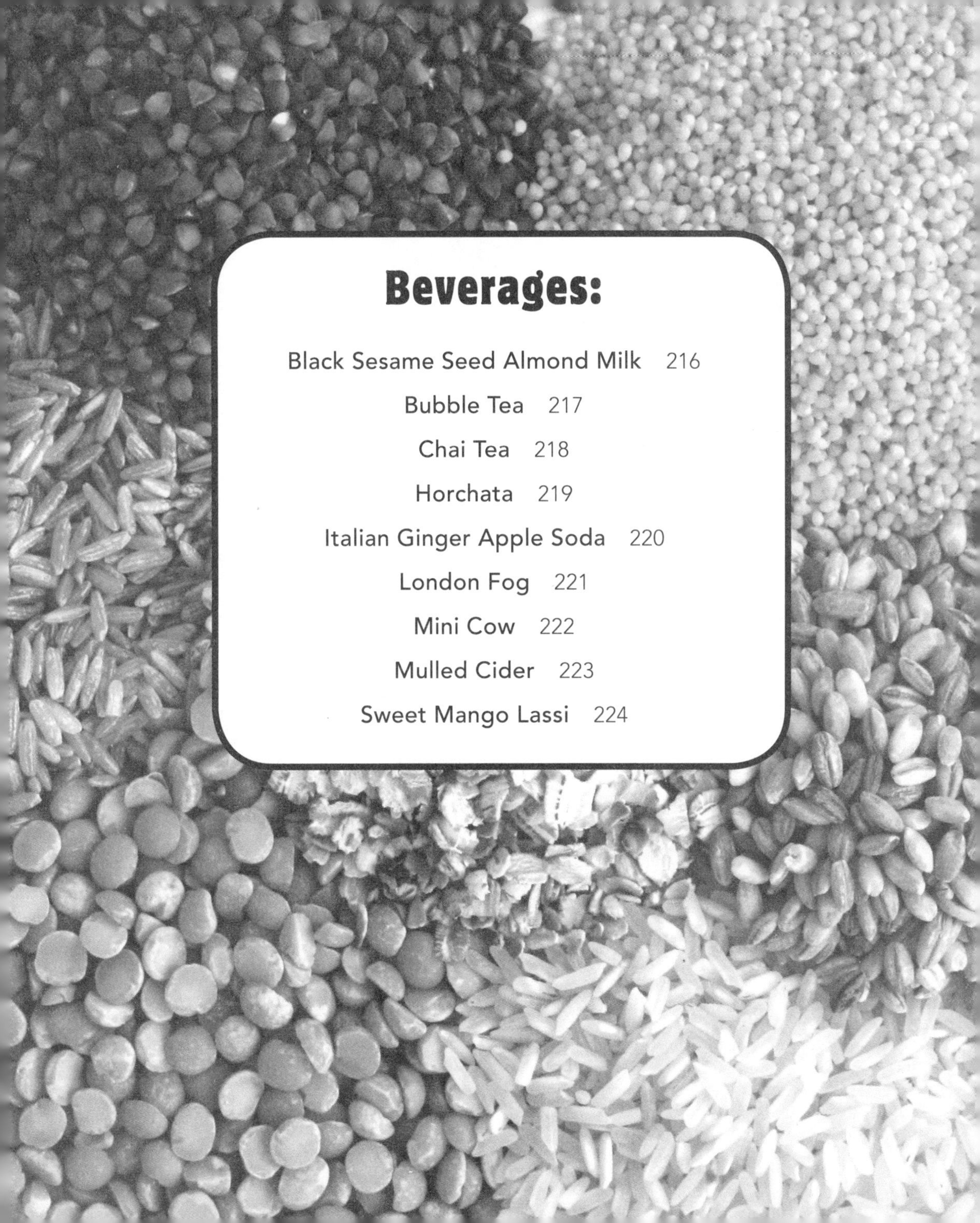

Beverages:

Thailand

Black Sesame Seed Almond Milk

Serve hot or cold.

Yield: 2 servings

¼ cup black sesame seeds

2 cups unsweetened almond milk

12 pitted dates, chopped

Sweetener to taste

In food mill, grind sesame seeds.

In a blender, blend sesame seeds, almond milk, and dates until smooth.

Add sweetener to taste.

Heat if preferred.

Bubble Tea

Bubble tea is served chilled and contains large whole tapioca pearls.

Yield: 8 servings

- **¾ cup large pearl tapioca (often found in Asian specialty stores)**
- **8 black tea bags**
- **4 cups water**
- **¼ cup sugar**
- **¼ cup brown sugar**
- **½ cup water**
- **4 cups cold soy milk**
- **Ice cubes**

Boil tapioca in at least eight cups of water, stirring occasionally, until the tapioca pearls become clear (you may need to change out the water and continue to cook the tapioca if the water becomes too cloudy and starchy).

Drain and rinse tapioca. Place tapioca pearls in cold water and refrigerate until needed.

Boil four cups water and remove from heat. Add tea and steep for five minutes. Discard tea bags. Chill tea until needed.

In a small sauce pan, combine sugar, brown sugar, and ½ cup water. Bring to a boil, reduce heat to low and simmer for one minute. Chill this syrup until needed.

In a glass, combine two Tbs. tapioca pearls, ½ cup tea, ½ cup soy milk, and 1½ Tbs. syrup. Add ice.

Chai Tea

Also known as Masala Chai, this tea was reserved for royalty five to nine thousand years ago.

Yield: 3 servings

1 whole vanilla bean

14 whole cardamom pods, lightly crushed

1 Tbs. diced ginger

2 3-inch cinnamon sticks

6 whole cloves

6 whole black peppercorns

2 cups water

2 cups soy milk

3 Darjeeling tea bags or other black tea

Sweetener to taste (brown sugar, stevia, etc.)

Split vanilla bean in half lengthwise. With a dinner knife, scrape out the pulp.

In a 3-quart saucepan, add the split vanilla bean and its pulp.

Add remaining ingredients except tea and sweetener.

Bring to a boil and reduce heat to low. Cover and simmer for 10 minutes.

Remove from heat.

Add tea bags and let steep for five minutes. Squeeze tea bags into liquid and then discard.

Strain tea through a fine strainer and discard spices.

Add sweetener to taste.

Reheat if needed.

Horchata

Horchata goes well with spicy foods and hot summer days.

Yield: 3 servings

½ cup long grain white rice

4 cups hot tap water

1 tsp. vanilla

¼ cup sugar

¼ tsp. cinnamon

Combine rice and hot tap water. Let sit for 30 minutes.

In a blender, blend rice, water, vanilla, sugar, and cinnamon for 30 seconds.

Strain, saving liquid and discarding rice.

Chill.

USA

Italian Ginger Apple Soda

Italian sodas were created in the USA despite its name.

Yield: 10 servings

2 cups chopped fresh unpeeled ginger

2 cups sugar

2 cups water

Juice of 1 lime

Juice of 1 lemon

8 cups sparkling apple cider

Ice cubes

Place ginger, sugar, water, lime juice, and lemon juice in a blender and blend for 10 seconds.

Place ginger mixture in a large pot. Bring to a boil, reduce heat to low, cover, and simmer for one hour.

Strain out the ginger, keeping the liquid and discarding the ginger.

Place ginger beer syrup in the refrigerator to chill.

To serve, pour ¼ cup of the syrup and ¾ cup sparkling apple cider into a glass over ice.

London Fog

Many fun variations of this beverage exist like the Oregon Mist which is made with green tea, the Seattle Fog which is made with hazelnut syrup, and the Dublin Fog which uses English Breakfast tea.

Yield: 1 cup

½ cup boiling water

1 Earl Grey tea bag

1 cup steamed or hot soy milk

2 Tbs. sugar*

1 tsp. vanilla*

** Substitute sugar and vanilla with one shot (2 Tbs.) vanilla syrup.*

Steep tea in hot water for five minutes.

Remove tea bag and add soy milk, sugar, and vanilla.

USA

Mini Cow

Yield: 2 servings

1½ cups vegan vanilla ice cream

12 oz. root beer

2 Tbs. chocolate syrup

Place all ingredients in a blender and blend until almost smooth.

Moo.

Mulled Cider

Yield: 4 servings

1 orange, quartered

12 whole cloves

4 cups apple juice/cider

2 Tbs. brown sugar

1 cinnamon stick

¼ tsp. nutmeg

In a 3-quart saucepan, combine all ingredients.

Cover and simmer for 60 minutes.

Lightly squeeze oranges.

Remove oranges, cloves, and cinnamon stick.

Serve hot.

India

Sweet Mango Lassi

Yield: 4 servings

2 cups plain vegan yogurt or 12 oz. firm silken tofu

8 oz. frozen mango chunks, or two fresh mangoes, peeled, pitted, and diced

1 cup water

¼ cup sugar

In a blender, blend all ingredients until smooth.

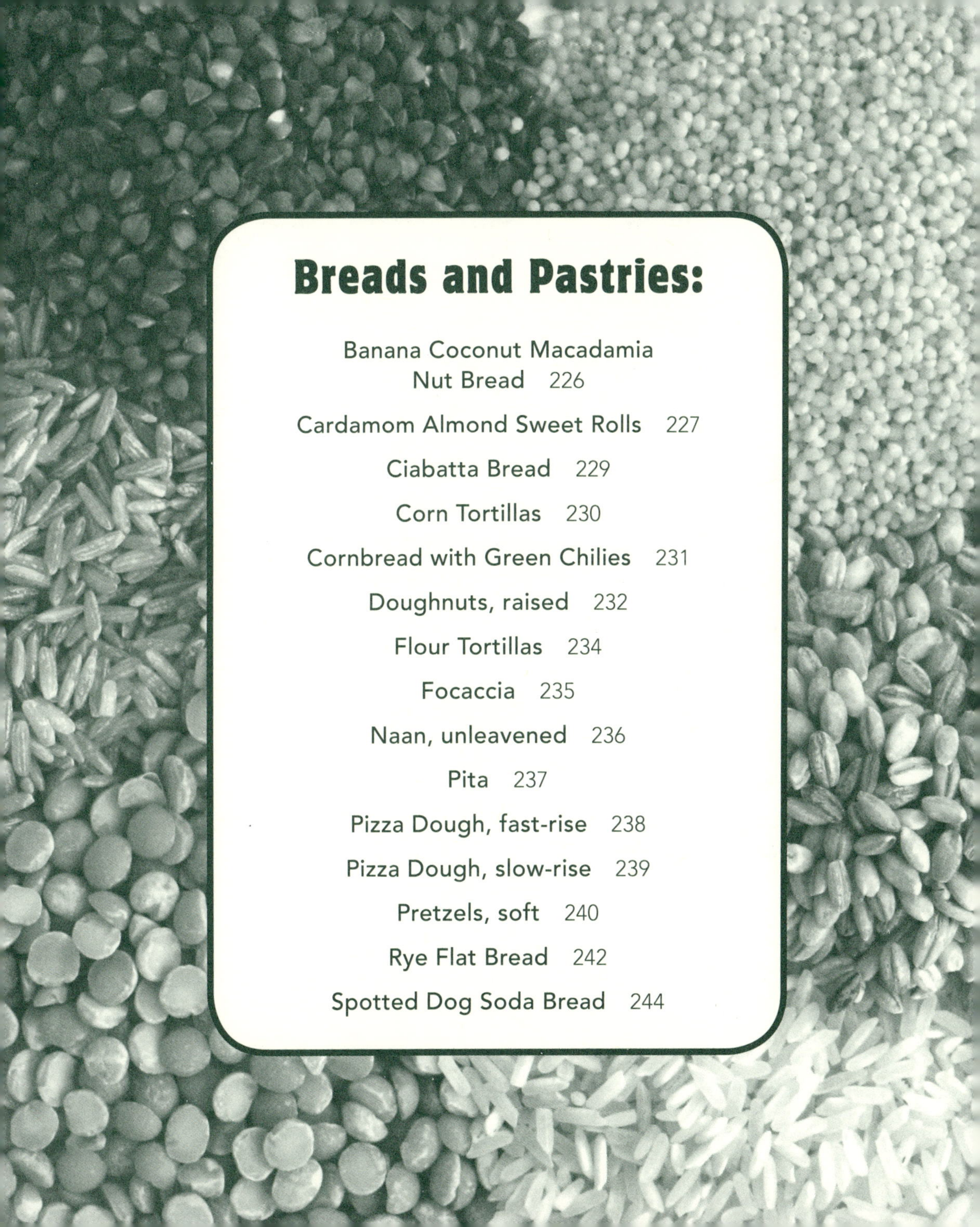

Breads and Pastries:

Hawaii, USA

Banana Coconut Macadamia Nut Bread

Yield: 2 loaves

4 cups flour*

1½ cups sugar

1 cup chopped macadamia nuts

2 tsp. baking powder

2 tsp. egg replacer powder

2 tsp. salt

1 tsp. baking soda

4 very ripe bananas, mashed

14-oz. can unsweetened coconut milk

1 Tbs. vanilla

Pan spray

* *Use part whole wheat flour if you prefer.*

Preheat oven to 350°F.

In a large bowl, whisk together the flour, sugar, macadamia nuts, baking powder, egg replacer powder, salt, and baking soda. Set aside.

In a blender, blend the mashed bananas, coconut milk, and vanilla.

With a spoon, combine flour mixture with banana mixture just until combined.

Divide batter between two pan-sprayed loaf pans.

Bake for one hour or until toothpick inserted in center comes out clean.

Cardamom Almond Sweet Rolls

Yield: 12 rolls

Rolls:

1 Tbs. active dry yeast (¼-oz. package)

1 tsp. sugar

¼ cup warm water (110°F)

6 oz. firm silken tofu

⅓ cup sugar

½ cup vegetable oil

½ cup soy milk

1 Tbs. vanilla

1 tsp. salt

3¼ cups flour*

Filling:

¼ cup vegan margarine, melted

1 cup brown sugar

¾ cup golden raisins

¾ cup sliced almonds

2 tsp. ground cardamom

2 tsp. cinnamon

** Use part whole wheat flour if you prefer.*

Rolls:

In a large bowl, whisk together the yeast, one tsp. sugar, and warm water. Let sit for 10 minutes.

In a blender, blend the tofu, ⅓ cup sugar, vegetable oil, soy milk, vanilla, and salt. Add to yeast mixture.

Add flour and stir just until combined.

On a floured surface, knead dough for seven minutes (if using an electric mixer to knead the dough, add an additional ¼ cup of flour and reduce kneading time to 5 minutes).

Place dough in a large oiled bowl.

Cover with clear wrap and let sit in a warm place until doubled in size, one to two hours.

Punch down dough and knead one minute.

On a floured surface, roll out dough to 12-inches × 16-inches.

Filling:

In a small bowl, combine filling ingredients.

Assembling Rolls:

Distribute filling mixture evenly on top of dough.

Roll up dough starting on the 12-inch edge.

Cut dough into 12 even pieces.

Place rolls in a lightly oiled 9-inch × 13-inch baking dish. Cover with clear wrap and let sit in a warm place until doubled in size, about 1 hour.

Preheat oven to 375°F.

Bake for 20 minutes or until center is no longer doughy.

Ciabatta Bread

Ciabatta means "slipper bread" in Italian.

Yield: 1 loaf

1¾ cups warm water (110°F)

1 Tbs. yeast (¼-oz. package)

3¼ cups flour*

1 Tbs. salt

** Use part whole wheat flour if you prefer.*

In a large bowl, whisk together the water and yeast.

Add flour and salt. Dough will be sticky.

Cover with clear wrap and let sit at room temperature for 12-24 hours. The longer it sits the more flavor it will have.

With a rubber spatula, stir dough for one minute.

Place dough on a floured surface, dust with flour, and cover with clear wrap.

Let sit at room temperature for two hours.

In a cold oven, place an empty 9-inch × 13-inch baking dish.

Preheat oven to 450°F.

After oven is preheated, remove baking dish and add dough (do not oil dish).

Cover with a tight-fitting dome lid or a tight-fitting dome of foil, leaving enough room for bread to expand.

Bake for 30 minutes.

Remove cover and continue baking for 15 more minutes or until loaf is lightly browned.

Mexico

Corn Tortillas

Making corn tortillas is a bit of an art. Subtle adjustments on the amount of liquid and cooking times may be needed.

Yield: 16 6-inch tortillas

2 cups masa flour

½ tsp. salt

1¼ cups water

Waxed or parchment paper

In a bowl, combine masa and salt.

Stir in water.

Mix dough for two minutes (using your hands works well for this step).

Divide dough into 16 dough balls.

Place a dough ball between two pieces of waxed or parchment paper. Using a tortilla press or a rolling pin, press or roll dough into a 6-inch round.

On a medium-hot (400°F) dry griddle, grill tortilla for one minute on each side or until cooked.

Repeat with remaining dough.

Cornbread with Green Chilies

Yield: 9 pieces

1¼ cups cornmeal

¾ cup flour

¼ cup sugar

2 tsp. baking powder

2 tsp. egg replacer powder

1 tsp. salt

7-oz. can diced green chilies

1 cup unsweetened soy milk

⅓ cup vegetable oil

Preheat oven to 400°F.

In a large bowl, combine dry ingredients.

Whisk in the green chilies, soy milk, and vegetable oil.

Pour batter into an oiled 8-inch × 8-inch baking dish.

Bake for 25 minutes or until toothpick inserted in the center comes out clean.

Doughnuts, raised

Yield: 12 doughnuts, plus doughnut holes!

1 Tbs. active dry yeast (¼-oz. package)

1 tsp. sugar

¼ cup warm water (110°F)

6 oz. firm silken tofu

½ cup sugar

½ cup vegetable oil

½ cup soy milk

1 Tbs. vanilla

1 tsp. salt

3¾ cups flour

Vanilla Glaze (pg. 338)

Vegetable oil for frying, about 48 oz.

In a large bowl, whisk together the yeast, one tsp. sugar, and warm water. Let sit for 10 minutes.

In a blender, blend the tofu, ½ cup sugar, ½ cup vegetable oil, soy milk, vanilla, and salt.

Add contents of the blender to the contents of the large bowl and mix just until combined.

Add flour and stir until combined.

On a floured surface, knead dough for seven minutes (if using an electric mixer to knead the dough, add an additional ¼ cup of flour and reduce kneading time to 5 minutes).

Place kneaded dough in a large oiled bowl, cover with clear wrap, and let sit in a warm place until doubled in size, one to two hours.

Punch down dough and knead for one minute.

On a floured surface, roll out dough to 10-inches × 12-inches.

Cut out doughnuts with doughnut cutter. You can also divide dough into 12 pieces and hand-form each piece into a doughnut.

Place doughnuts on a floured surface. Dust top of doughnuts with flour, cover with clear wrap, and let rise for 20 minutes.

Meanwhile, prepare vanilla glaze and set aside.

Heat one inch of oil in a large, heavy bottom skillet.

Using a candy thermometer, heat oil to 350°F. Regulate heat while cooking to maintain a temperature range of 340-360°F.

In batches, add doughnuts to oil and fry until browned on each side and cooked in the middle, about one minute per side.

Place on cooling rack for five minutes.

Brush with Vanilla Glaze.

Variation: Maple Bars

Form doughnuts in a bar shape. Once fried, top with Maple Frosting (pg. 328).

Mexico

Flour Tortillas

Flour tortillas are traditionally unleavened flat bread, but over the years we've become accustomed to a lighter tortilla which contains a small amount of baking powder.

Yield: Six 8-inch tortillas

2 cups flour*

1 tsp. salt

¼ tsp. baking powder

1 Tbs. vegetable oil

¾ cup warm water

Vegetable oil for brushing

* *Use part whole wheat if preferred. Add one Tbs. additional water for every cup of whole wheat used.*

In a large bowl, combine flour, salt, and baking powder.

Stir in oil and water.

On a floured surface, knead dough for three minutes.

Cover and let rest for five minutes.

Divide dough into six balls.

Roll each ball into an 8-inch round.

Preheat electric griddle or skillet to 425°F, or put on medium-high heat if using a stovetop griddle or skillet.

Lightly oil tops of tortillas.

Place tortillas, oiled side down, on griddle or frying pan and lightly oil second side.

Grill tortillas for one minute on each side or until done.

Focaccia

Yield: One 15-inch X 10-inch loaf

1 Tbs. yeast (¼-oz. package)

1¼ cups warm water (110°F)

½ tsp. sugar

3¼ cups bread flour*, divided

¼ cup olive oil

1 Tbs. salt

¼ cup chopped fresh basil leaves

1 tsp garlic powder

½ tsp. salt

Olive oil for brushing

** Use part whole wheat flour if preferred.*

In a large bowl, whisk together the yeast, water, and sugar. Let sit for 10 minutes.

Whisk in one cup of the flour and ¼ cup olive oil.

Cover with clear wrap.

Let sit for 24 hours at room temperature.

With a spoon, stir in 1 Tbs. salt and the remaining 2¼ cups flour.

On a floured surface, knead dough for eight minutes (if using an electric mixer to knead the dough, add an additional ¼ cup of flour and reduce kneading time to 5 minutes).

Cover and let dough rest for five minutes.

Press into an oiled 15-inch × 10-inch baking dish.

Sprinkle with basil, garlic powder, and ½ tsp. salt. Brush with olive oil.

Dimple top of dough with fingers.

Cover.

Let rise until doubled in size, about 50 minutes.

Preheat oven to 400°F.

Uncover and bake until no longer doughy, about 17 minutes.

Naan, unleavened

Yield: Eight 6-inch breads

½ cup uncooked bulgur

2 tsp. salt

3 Tbs. olive oil

¾ cup boiling water

1½ cups flour*

Olive oil for brushing (optional)

** Use part whole wheat flour if preferred.*

In a large bowl, combine bulgur, salt, oil, and boiling water. Let sit for 15 minutes.

Stir in flour.

On a floured surface, knead dough for five minutes.

Cover and let rest for five minutes.

Divide dough into eight pieces and form into balls.

On a lightly floured surface, roll each ball into a 6-inch round.

Preheat griddle to 400°F or medium-high heat.

Grill one minute on each side or until done.

Brush the tops of the cooked Naan with additional olive oil if preferred.

Pita

This is simply flat bread, not the pita with pockets that you find in the grocery store.

Yield: 8 pitas

1 Tbs. active dry yeast (¼-oz. package)

1½ cups warm water (110°F)

2 Tbs. olive oil

2 tsp. salt

3½ cups flour*

** Use part whole wheat flour if preferred.*

In a large bowl, whisk together the yeast and water. Let sit for 10 minutes.

Whisk in oil and salt.

Stir in flour.

On a floured surface, knead dough for seven minutes.

Cover dough and let rise until doubled in size, about one hour.

Punch down dough and knead for one minute.

Divide dough into eight pieces and form into balls.

Roll each ball into an 8-inch round.

Preheat griddle to 400°F or medium heat with a skillet.

Grill for one minute on each side or until done.

Pizza Dough, fast-rise

Yield: One 14-inch thick-crust or two 14-inch thin-crusts

1 Tbs. active dry yeast (¼-oz. package)

1 cup warm water (110°F)

1 tsp. sugar

2½ cups flour*

1 tsp. salt

¼ cup olive oil

** Use part whole wheat flour if you prefer.*

In a large bowl, whisk together the yeast, water, and sugar. Let sit for 10 minutes.

Stir in flour.

On a floured surface, knead dough for seven minutes (if using an electric mixer to knead the dough, add an additional ¼ cup of flour and reduce kneading time to 5 minutes).

Place dough in an oiled bowl and cover with clear wrap. Let sit until doubled in size, about one hour.

Punch down dough and knead for one minute.

Let dough rest for five minutes.

Use dough as desired.

Pizza Dough, slow-rise

Yield: One 14-inch pizza crust

The dough for this crust must ferment for 24 hours.

1 Tbs. yeast (¼-oz. package)

¾ cup warm water (110°F)

½ tsp. sugar

1½ cups bread flour*, divided

2 Tbs. olive oil

1½ tsp. salt

Additional flour for kneading

** Use part whole wheat flour if preferred.*

In a large bowl, whisk together the yeast, water, and sugar. Let sit for 10 minutes.

Whisk in ¾ cup of the flour and olive oil.

Place in a large bowl leaving enough room for dough to triple in size.

Cover with clear wrap and let ferment for 24 hours at room temperature.

With a spoon, stir in salt and the remaining ¾ cup flour.

On a floured surface, knead dough for 10 minutes (if using an electric mixer to knead the dough, add an additional ¼ cup of flour and reduce kneading time to 5 minutes).

Place dough in an oiled bowl, cover, and let rise until doubled in size, about 1½ hours.

Punch down dough and knead for 10 seconds.

Cover and let rest for five minutes.

Use as desired.

Germany

Pretzels, soft

Yield: 8

1 Tbs. active dry yeast (¼-oz. package)

1 tsp. sugar

1 cup warm water (110°F)

2 Tbs. vegetable oil

2¼ cups flour*

1½ tsp. salt

Coarse salt (to taste)

** Use part whole wheat flour if you prefer.*

In a large bowl, whisk together the yeast, sugar, warm water, and oil. Let sit for 10 minutes.

With a spoon, add flour and 1½ tsp. salt.

On a floured surface, knead dough for seven minutes (if using an electric mixer to knead the dough, add an additional ¼ cup of flour and reduce kneading time to 5 minutes).

Cover dough and let rest for five minutes.

Divide dough into eight pieces.

Roll each piece into a 16-inch rope.

Twist ropes into pretzel shapes: Make a U shape, twist loose ends once around each other, take loose ends and bring down the middle area of the U and press into dough.

Place pretzels on a floured surface and dust tops lightly with flour.

Cover and let rise for 30 minutes.

Bring a large pan of water to a boil, preheat oven to 475°F, and oil a large baking sheet.

In batches, boil pretzels for one minute on each side.

Pretzels, soft
(*continued*)

Transfer pretzels to the oiled baking sheet and sprinkle with desired amount of salt.

Bake until browned and cooked in the middle, about 10 minutes.

Rye Flat Bread

Yield: 12 6-inch flat breads

1 cup boiling water

¼ cup bulgur

Zest of 1 orange

Juice of 1 orange

2 Tbs. molasses

1 Tbs. active dry yeast (¼-oz. package)

2 Tbs. vegetable oil

1½ cups dark rye flour

1¼ cups flour

1 tsp. salt

1 Tbs. lightly ground caraway seeds

Olive oil for brushing

In a large bowl, combine boiling water, bulgur, orange zest, and orange juice. Let sit for 30 minutes.

Add molasses, yeast, and vegetable oil. Let sit for 10 minutes.

It a separate bowl, combine rye flour, flour, salt, and caraway seeds.

Add yeast mixture to flour mixture and mix just until combined.

On a floured surface, knead dough for seven minutes (if using an electric mixer to knead the dough, add an additional ¼ cup of flour and reduce kneading time to 5 minutes).

Place kneaded dough in a large oiled bowl, cover with clear wrap, and let sit in a warm place until doubled in size, about 1 hour.

Punch down dough and knead for one minute.

Divide dough into 12 pieces.

On a lightly floured surface, roll each piece into a 6-inch round.

Preheat griddle to 400°F or medium-high heat.

Grill one minute on each side or until done.

Brush the tops of the cooked rye bread with olive oil after removing from griddle.

Ireland

Spotted Dog Soda Bread

Spotted Dog is Irish Soda Bread, which contains currants or raisins.

Yield: 12 servings

2¾ cups flour*

½ cup sugar

2 tsp. baking powder

1 tsp. salt

½ tsp. baking soda

½ cup currants or raisins

½ cup vegan margarine, melted

¾ cup firm silken tofu

¾ cup soy milk

1 tsp. vinegar

* *Use part whole wheat flour if you prefer.*

Preheat oven to 425°F.

In a large bowl, whisk together the flour, sugar, baking powder, salt, baking soda, and currants or raisins.

In a blender, blend the margarine, tofu, soy milk, and vinegar.

Add blended ingredients to flour mixture and stir just until combined.

Place dough on a lightly oiled baking sheet and form into a rounded loaf.

Cut a traditional × on the top.

Bake for 20 minutes or until toothpick inserted in center comes out clean.

Desserts:

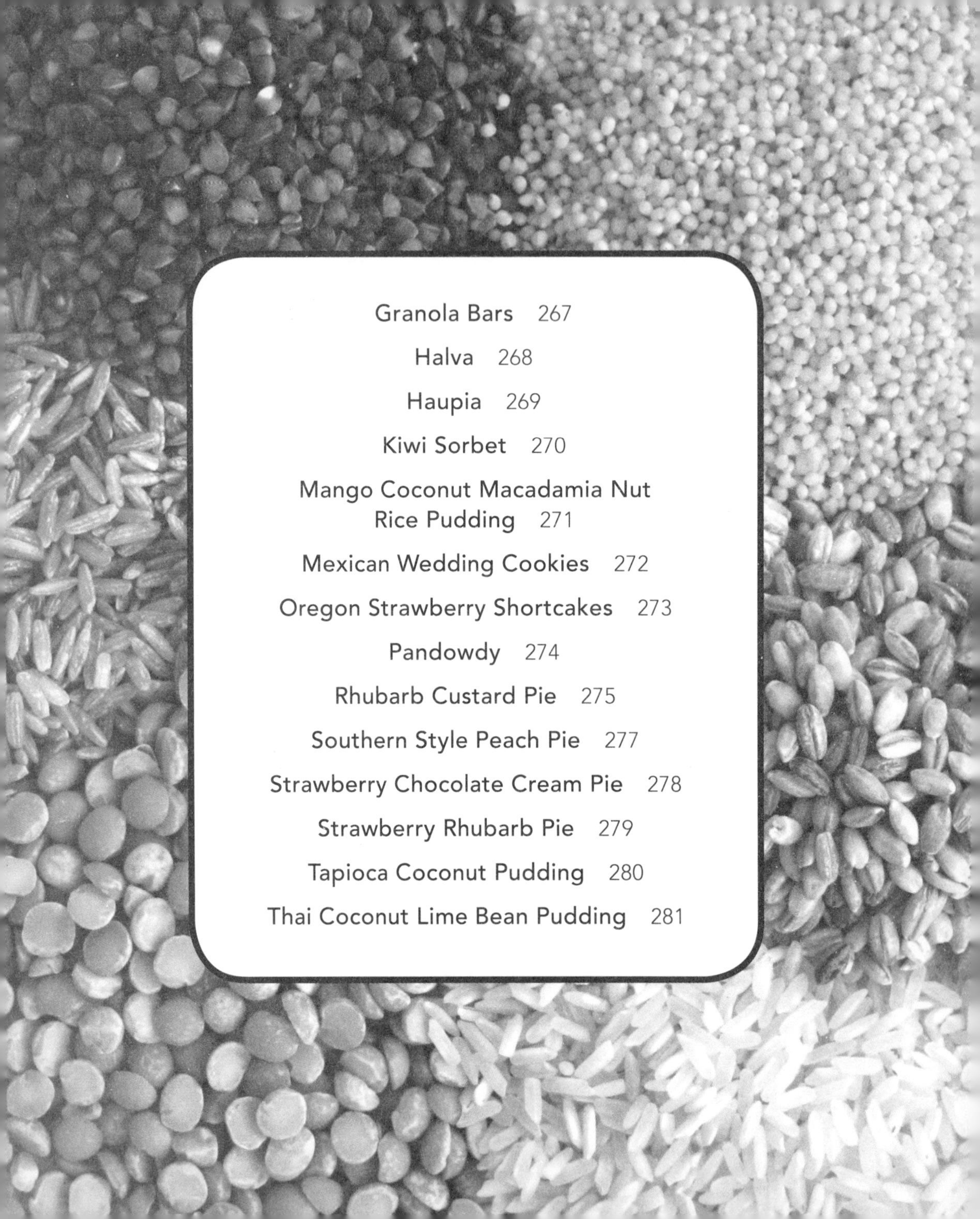

Almond Butter Chocolate Cheese Cake, no bake

Yield: One 9-inch pie

9-inch Graham Cracker Crust (pg. 333)

½ cup sugar

2 Tbs. cornstarch

¾ cup canned unsweetened light coconut milk

3 oz. semisweet vegan baking chocolate, chopped

1 cup creamy almond butter

2 8-oz containers vegan cream cheese

Prepare graham cracker crust and set aside.

In a small bowl, whisk together the sugar and cornstarch until fully combined.

In a 3-quart saucepan, combine coconut milk with sugar/cornstarch mixture. Heat until thickened, whisking often.

Remove from heat and whisk in chocolate until smooth.

Whisk in almond butter, until smooth.

With an electric mixer, mix in cream cheese until smooth.

Scoop into prepared crust and smooth top.

Chill until set.

France

Apple and Baguette Bread Pudding

Yield: 8 servings

4 cups soy milk

2 green apples, peeled, cored, and small dice

½ cup sugar

¼ cup brown sugar

1 Tbs. vanilla

1 tsp. cinnamon

⅛ tsp. nutmeg

16-oz. baguette, large dice

Whipped Cream (pg. 339) (optional)

Preheat oven to 325°F.

In a large bowl, whisk together the soy milk, diced apples, sugars, vanilla, cinnamon, and nutmeg.

Stir in diced baguette and let sit for 10 minutes.

Pour into a lightly oiled 9-inch × 13-inch baking dish.

Bake for 35 minutes.

Serve warm.

Top with Whipped Cream if preferred.

Apple Strudel

Yield: 8 servings

1 sheet vegan puff pastry, thawed

3 green apples

Zest of one lemon, minced

½ cup sliced almonds

¼ cup brown sugar

2 Tbs. soy milk

2 Tbs. flour

¼ tsp. cinnamon

1 Tbs. soy milk

1 Tbs. vegetable oil

Powdered sugar (optional)

Peel, quarter, and core apples. Slice into ⅛-inch slices. Place sliced apples into a large bowl.

Stir in the lemon zest, almonds, brown sugar, 2 Tbs. soy milk, flour, and cinnamon. Set aside.

On a floured surface, roll out the puff pastry sheet to 12-inches × 16-inches.

With the 12-inch side parallel to the counter edge, spoon the apple mixture onto the bottom ¾ of the puff pastry, staying one inch away from the edge.

Roll up puff pastry starting on the apple-covered end. Place on an oiled baking sheet seam side down.

Tuck pastry ends under.

Combine the one Tbs. soy milk and oil and brush top of strudel.

Score top of strudel.

Preheat oven to 375°F.

Bake for 40 minutes.

Cool at room temperature for 20 minutes before serving.

Dust with powdered sugar if desired.

Arroz Con Leche

Yield: 6 servings

1 cup white basmati rice, rinsed

1½ cups water

14-oz. can unsweetened light coconut milk

Zest of one lemon, minced

1 vanilla bean or 2 tsp. vanilla extract

¼ cup sugar

¼ cup golden raisins

⅛ tsp. salt

In a 3-quart saucepan, bring rice and water to a boil.

Reduce heat to low, cover, and simmer for 20 minutes or until rice is tender.

Split vanilla bean in half lengthwise and scrape out the pulp to be added in next step.

Add remaining ingredients.

Bring to a low boil.

Simmer for five minutes, stirring occasionally.

Serve warm or chilled.

Blackberry Pie

Yield: One 9-inch pie

2 quarts fresh blackberries

½ cup sugar

2 Tbs. lemon juice

2 Tbs. cornstarch

2 Tbs. flour

2 tsp. vegan margarine

9-inch Double Pie Crust (pg. 332)

In a large bowl, combine blackberries, sugar, lemon juice, cornstarch, and flour.

Prepare pie crust. Line bottom of pie dish with bottom crust.

Preheat oven to 400°F.

Pour blackberry filling into pie dish.

Dot top of filling with the margarine.

Cover with top crust and seal edges.

With a dinner knife, pierce the top crust a few times to allow steam to escape.

Bake for 40 minutes or until juice begins to bubble.

New England, USA

Blueberry Buckle

Yield: 12 servings

3 cups flour*

1 cup sugar

1 tsp. cinnamon

½ tsp. nutmeg

½ tsp. allspice

½ tsp. salt

¾ cup vegetable oil

1 cup soy milk

1 cup fresh or frozen blueberries

1 Tbs. baking powder

* *Use part whole wheat if preferred*

Preheat oven to 375°F.

In a large bowl, whisk together the flour, sugar, cinnamon, nutmeg, allspice, and salt.

Using a fork, mix in the oil until the mixture looks like crumb topping.

Reserve 1½ cups of this mixture to be used later for the topping.

To the non-reserved mixture, add the soy milk, blueberries, and baking powder (to make the batter) just until combined.

Spread batter into an oiled 9-inch × 13-inch baking dish.

Sprinkle the 1½ cups reserved topping on the top of the batter.

Bake for 25 minutes or until toothpick inserted in center comes out clean.

Hillsboro, Oregon, USA

Blueberry Bon Bons

I was inspired to make these summertime treats by the local blueberries sold at the farmers market in Orenco Station, Hillsboro, OR.

Yield: 20 cookies

20 large fresh blueberries

½ cup vegan margarine

¾ cup powdered sugar

1 Tbs. vanilla

1 Tbs. soy milk

⅛ tsp. salt

1½ cups all-purpose flour

By hand, food processor, or mixer, combine the margarine, powdered sugar, vanilla, soy milk, and salt until smooth.

Place in a bowl and stir in flour.

Hand-roll dough into twenty, ¾-inch balls.

Press your thumb into the center of the cookie to create an indention for a blueberry.

Place one blueberry in center and work dough back into a ball around the blueberry.

Place on an ungreased cookie sheet.

Preheat oven to 350°F.

Bake for 15 minutes, or until lightly browned on the bottom.

USA

Blueberry Pie

Yield: One 9-inch pie

5 cups fresh blueberries, or 5 cups frozen blueberries, thawed

¾ cup sugar

3 Tbs. cornstarch

⅛ tsp. salt

¼ cup cold water

1 Tbs. lemon juice

1 Tbs. vegan margarine

Double Pie Crust (pg. 332)

1 tsp. sugar

In a small bowl combine ¾ cup sugar, cornstarch, salt, and water.

Place blueberries in a 3-quart saucepan. Add sugar mixture.

Cook on medium heat until mixture comes to a boil, stirring constantly.

Add lemon juice and margarine.

Prepare pie crusts. Line bottom of pie dish with bottom crust.

Pour blueberries into pie dish.

Cover with top crust and seal edges.

Sprinkle the top of the pie with the one tsp. of sugar.

With a dinner knife, pierce the top crust a few times to allow steam to escape.

Bake in a preheated 425°F oven for 35 minutes or until lightly browned.

Butterscotch Pudding

Yield: 4 servings

¼ cup vegan margarine

¾ cup dark brown sugar

2¾ cups cold soy milk

¼ cup cornstarch

1½ tsp. vanilla

¼ tsp. salt

In a 3-quart saucepan, melt margarine with brown sugar.

In a medium bowl, combine soy milk, cornstarch, vanilla, and salt.

Whisk into margarine mixture.

Bring to a boil, whisking constantly.

Pour into a 9-inch × 13-inch dish.

Refrigerate until chilled and set, stirring occasionally.

Cardamom Coconut Bread Pudding

Yield: 8 servings

2 14-oz. cans unsweetened coconut milk

1 cup soy milk

½ cup golden raisins

½ cup shelled pistachios

½ cup sugar

¼ cup brown sugar

1 Tbs. vanilla

1 tsp. ground cardamom

½ tsp. cinnamon

16-oz. baguette, large dice

Whipped Cream (pg. 339) (optional)

Preheat oven to 325°F.

In a large bowl, whisk together all ingredients except baguette.

Stir in baguette and let sit for 10 minutes.

Pour into a 9-inch × 13-inch baking dish.

Bake for 35 minutes.

Serve warm with Whipped Cream if desired.

Carrot Cake

Yield: Two 9-inch rounds or one 9-inch X 13-inch cake

2½ cups flour

1½ cups sugar

1 Tbs. baking powder

2 tsp. baking soda

1 tsp. cornstarch

1 tsp. salt

1½ tsp. cinnamon

½ tsp. nutmeg

1½ cups soy milk

¾ cup vegetable oil

1 Tbs. vanilla

1 cup shredded carrots

½ cup chopped walnuts

½ cup raisins

Cream Cheese Frosting (pg. 326)

Preheat oven to 350°F.

Oil and flour pan(s) or line bottom(s) with parchment paper.

In a large bowl, whisk together the flour, sugar, baking powder, baking soda, cornstarch, salt, cinnamon, and nutmeg.

Add the soy milk, vegetable oil, and vanilla. With an electric mixer, mix on low speed just until combined. Turn mixer to high and mix two more minutes, scraping edges of bowl occasionally.

Stir in the carrots, walnuts, and raisins.

Pour batter into prepared pan(s).

Bake for 35 minutes, or until toothpick inserted in the center comes out clean.

Cool at room temperature for 10 minutes. Remove from pan(s) and place on a wire cooling rack. Cool completely before frosting.

Chai Tapioca Pudding

Yield: 5 servings

Good with Whipped Cream (pg. 339)

½ cup small pearl tapioca

1 cup brewed black tea

2½ cups soy milk

1 Tbs. vanilla

¾ cup brown sugar

¼ tsp. ground cardamom

¼ tsp. ground ginger

⅛ tsp. cinnamon

In a 3-quart saucepan, combine all ingredients and let sit for 30 minutes.

Bring to a boil, reduce heat to low, and simmer until tapioca pearls are clear (about 20 minutes), stirring frequently.

Pour into a container and refrigerate until chilled.

Chocolate Fondue

Fondue has its roots in Switzerland with cheese fondues. You can add liqueurs or extracts to your fondue if you wish.

Yield: 1 cup

3 oz. semisweet vegan baking chocolate squares, chopped

⅔ cup canned unsweetened light coconut milk

Dipping Options:

Fruit or Fruit Kabobs (strawberries, pineapple, banana, apple, blueberries, kiwi)

Brownies

Sponge or Pound Cake

Ginger Bread Cookies

Chocolate Chip Cookies

Sugar Cookies

Peanut Butter Cookies

Banana Bread

Zucchini Bread

Vegan Marshmallows

Crystallized Ginger

Dried Fruit (figs, plums, and apricots)

Nuts

Place chocolate in a medium bowl and set aside.

Bring coconut milk to a boil.

Pour over chocolate and let sit for five minutes.

Whisk until smooth.

Place in fondue pot.

France

Chocolate Mousse, or "Mousse au Chocolat"

Yield: 8 servings

2 14-oz. cans unsweetened and regular fat coconut milk, chilled overnight in refrigerator

4 oz. unsweetened chocolate baking squares, chopped

2 Tbs. vegetable oil

12 oz. extra firm silken tofu

1½ cups powdered sugar

½ tsp. salt

Chill cans of coconut milk overnight to solidify the coconut cream.

In a double boiler, melt chocolate with vegetable oil. Remove from heat until needed.

Pierce bottoms of coconut milk cans with a pointed can opener and drain off the liquid part (leaving thick coconut cream in can).

Open top of coconut milk cans and spoon the solidified coconut cream into a food processor.

Whip coconut cream with S blade until fluffy, about one minute.

Add silken tofu, powdered sugar, salt, and melted chocolate.

Process until smooth (about one minute), scraping sides as needed.

Chill a minimum of three hours.

Pipe or spoon into individual serving dishes.

Chocolate Peanut Butter Coconut Truffles

Yield: 20

½ cup vegan chocolate chips

½ cup chopped peanuts

¼ cup golden raisins

¼ cup peanut butter

1 cup sweetened shredded coconut, chopped

In a food processor, process chocolate chips, peanuts, and raisins until smooth.

Add peanut butter and process just until combined.

Remove mixture from food processor and place in a bowl.

Roll mixture into small, walnut-sized balls.

Roll balls in shredded coconut until well coated.

Chill until served.

Coconut Mango Pudding

Yield: 6 servings

½ cup sugar

¼ cup cornstarch

3 cups frozen mango chunks, lightly thawed

2 14-oz. cans unsweetened coconut milk

In a small bowl whisk together the sugar and cornstarch and set aside.

In a blender, blend mangos and coconut milk until smooth.

Transfer mango mixture to a 3-quart saucepan. Bring to a boil, stirring frequently.

Slowly whisk sugar and cornstarch mixture into the mango mixture.

Cook until thickened, stirring constantly.

Chill until set.

Crème Brulee

One trick to melting the sugar to form the Crème Brulee crust is to go over it a second time with the torch to evenly melt the sugar to create a nice dark brown color.

Yield: 5 servings

14-oz. can light unsweetened coconut milk*

½ cup soy milk

⅓ cup sugar

2 Tbs. brown sugar

3 Tbs. flour

5 tsp. cornstarch

½ tsp. salt

1 whole vanilla bean

5 tsp. sugar

In a blender, add the coconut milk, soy milk, ⅓ cup sugar, brown sugar, flour, cornstarch, and salt.

Split vanilla bean in half lengthwise. With a dinner knife, scrape out the pulp. Add pulp to the blender.

On low speed, blend until smooth, about 20 seconds.

Pour into a 3-quart saucepan. Bring to a boil, whisking constantly.

Pour thickened mixture into five ramekins or pan-sprayed muffin pan cups (without paper liners).

Chill in refrigerator until set, about four hours.

Sprinkle one tsp. of sugar evenly over each Crème Brulee.

Using a torch, melt the sugar to form a crisp and nearly-burnt top. You can also use the broiler setting in your oven if you are careful (because it can burn quickly).

Serve within 30 minutes (otherwise the crisp sugar topping will dissolve).

** If using regular coconut milk, reduce cornstarch to 4½ tsp.*

Dutch Apple Pie

Yield: One 9-inch pie

Crumb topping:

1½ cups flour

⅓ cup vegetable oil

⅓ cup brown sugar

¾ tsp. salt

Pie filling:

6 tart apples (peeled, cored, and sliced)

¾ cup sugar

2 Tbs. cornstarch

1 Tbs. lemon juice

1 tsp. cinnamon

1 9-inch Single Pie Crust (pg. 334)

Preheat oven to 375°F.

Crumb topping:

In a bowl, combine flour, oil, brown sugar, and salt. Set aside.

Pie filling:

In a separate bowl, combine apples, sugar, cornstarch, lemon juice, and cinnamon.

Assembling pie:

Prepare pie crust. Line bottom of pie dish with pie crust.

Pour apple mixture into pie dish.

Sprinkle crumb topping on top of apple mixture.

Bake until apples are tender, about 45-55 minutes. Cover crumb topping with foil if it becomes too brown before the apples are done cooking.

Fried Yellow Plantains

Yield: 4 servings

6 Tbs. sugar

1 tsp. cinnamon

2 cups water

¼ cup salt

2 yellow plantain bananas

Vegetable oil for frying

In a bowl, combine sugar and cinnamon and set aside.

In a second bowl, whisk together water and salt. Set aside.

Peel plantains and cut into ½-inch thick diagonal slices.

Preheat oil in large skillet. Grill plantains with oil until browned, about two minutes on each side.

Place fried plantains in salt water for one minute.

Remove plantains and pat dry with paper towels.

On a cutting board and using the palm of your hand, slightly squash plantains to ¼-inch thick.

In the large skillet, re-grill plantains with oil for an additional two minutes on each side, reusing the same oil.

Remove plantains from oil and toss with cinnamon and sugar. Serve warm.

Gooseberry Cobbler

Yield: 4 servings

Filling:

4 cups fresh gooseberries, or 4 cups frozen gooseberries, thawed

½ cup water

¾ cup sugar

3 Tbs. cornstarch

¼ tsp. cinnamon

Dumpling:

2 cups flour

2 Tbs. sugar

2½ tsp. baking powder

1 tsp. salt

1 cup soy milk

⅓ cup vegetable oil

Preheat oven to 375°F.

Filling:

In a large bowl, combine gooseberries, water, ½ cup sugar, cornstarch, and cinnamon. Transfer to an 8-inch × 8-inch baking dish.

Dumpling:

In a second large bowl, whisk together the flour, two Tbs. sugar, baking powder, and salt. With a spoon, stir in the soy milk and oil just until combined.

Assembling cobbler:

Drop eight dumplings onto the top of the gooseberry mixture.

Bake for 45 minutes or until dumplings are fully cooked.

Granola Bars

Yield: 16

1 cup water

¼ cup ground flax seeds

2 cups quick oatmeal, uncooked

1½ cups dried fruit (raisins, dates, cranberries, mango, banana, blueberry, etc.)

1 cup sliced or chopped nuts (almonds, walnuts, pecans, cashews, peanuts, etc.)

1 cup unsweetened coconut flakes

1 cup whole wheat flour

½ tsp. salt

Pan spray

1 cup nut butter (almond, peanut, etc.)

½ cup brown sugar

1 Tbs. vanilla

Preheat oven to 350°F.

In a 2-quart saucepan, bring water to a boil. Remove from heat and stir in flax seeds. Let sit for 10 minutes. Pour into a large bowl.

Add oatmeal, fruit, nuts, coconut flakes, flour, and salt. Mix and set aside.

In a separate bowl, whisk together the nut butter, brown sugar, and vanilla.

Combine nut butter mixture with oatmeal mixture.

Press into a 9-inch × 13-inch pan-sprayed baking dish.

Bake for 20 minutes.

Halva

Halva is popular in Africa, Asia, and Europe. The exact origin is unclear. The two types of halva are flour based and sesame seed/nut-butter based.

Yield: 12 pieces

1¾ cups tahini (16 oz.)

1½ tsp. vanilla

1 cup shelled whole pistachios, toasted

1½ cups sugar

½ cup water

1 Tbs. lime juice

Parchment paper

Line a loaf pan with parchment paper and set aside.

In a large bowl, combine tahini, vanilla, and pistachios. Set aside.

In a 2-quart saucepan with a candy thermometer attached, bring sugar, water, and lime juice to a boil.

Cook at a low boil until mixture reaches 250°F.

Slowly whisk the sugar water mixture into the tahini mixture.

Pour into the parchment-lined loaf pan.

Chill in refrigerator for one hour.

Cover.

Chill until set, about 12 hours.

Haupia

Yield: 6 servings

14-oz. can unsweetened coconut milk

1 cup soy milk

6 Tbs. cornstarch

⅓ cup sugar

In a 3-quart saucepan, whisk together all ingredients.

Heat until hot and thickened, stirring constantly.

Pour into an 8-inch × 8-inch baking dish.

Chill until set, about four hours (do not stir).

Dice into 1-inch squares.

Kiwi Sorbet

Yield: 10 servings

12 kiwis, peeled and quartered

¾ cup sugar

In a food processor, process kiwis and sugar until smooth.

Pour into a 9-inch × 13-inch baking dish and place in freezer.

With a metal spoon, stir sorbet (including the edges) every ten minutes until sorbet is completely frozen, about two hours.

Serve immediately for best results.

If served later, pull sorbet out of freezer 15 minutes before serving.

Mango Coconut Macadamia Nut Rice Pudding

Yield: 6 servings

1½ cups white jasmine rice, rinsed

2 cups water

14-oz. can unsweetened coconut milk

½ cup chopped macadamia nuts

½ cup chopped dried mango

¼ cup sugar

½ tsp. vanilla

½ tsp. salt

In a 3-quart saucepan, combine rice and water.

Let sit for 15 minutes.

Bring to a boil, reduce heat to low, cover, and simmer for 15 minutes or until rice is tender.

Add all remaining ingredients.

Slowly bring to a boil, stirring constantly.

Reduce heat to low and simmer for 10 minutes, stirring frequently.

Serve warm or chilled.

Mexican Wedding Cookies

Yield: 36

1 cup vegan margarine

¼ cup sugar

2 tsp. vanilla

2 cups flour

2 cups finely chopped pecans or walnuts

2 cups powdered sugar

Preheat oven to 400°F.

Cream together the margarine, ¼ cup sugar, and vanilla.

Stir in the flour and pecans or walnuts.

Roll into ¾-inch balls.

Place on an ungreased cookie sheet.

Bake until set but not brown, approximately 10-12 minutes.

Cool for five minutes.

Roll cookies in powdered sugar.

Once all cookies have been rolled in powdered sugar, roll them a second time in powdered sugar.

Oregon Strawberry Shortcakes

From living in Oregon, I've learned that this state prides itself in having the best strawberries in the world. These strawberries are mainly enjoyed by the locals because the berries have a high sugar content which makes them spoil quickly.

Yield: 8 servings

2 pints fresh strawberries (from Oregon if possible)

2 cups Whipped Cream (pg. 339)

Shortcake:

1¾ cups flour*

2 Tbs. sugar

1 Tbs. baking powder

1 tsp. salt

¾ cup soy milk

⅓ cup vegetable oil

** Substitute with half whole wheat flour if preferred.*

Preheat oven to 425°F.

Stem and slice strawberries. Place in refrigerator until needed.

Prepare Whipped Cream. Place in refrigerator until needed.

In a medium bowl, whisk together flour, sugar, baking powder, and salt.

Stir in the soy milk and oil just until combined.

Turn dough out onto a lightly floured surface and knead 5 times.

Roll out to ½-inch thick.

Cut into 8 pieces.

Place 1-inch apart on an ungreased baking sheet.

Bake for 13 minutes or until lightly browned and done in the middle.

While still warm, split cakes in half and top with Whipped Cream and strawberries.

New England, USA

Pandowdy

Yield: 6 servings

6 Granny Smith apples, peeled, cored, and ¼-inch sliced

⅓ cup maple syrup

Zest of one lemon, minced

Juice of one lemon

2 Tbs. cornstarch

Dough for a Single Pie Crust (pg. 334)

In a large bowl, combine apples, maple syrup, lemon zest, lemon juice, and cornstarch.

Pour into an 8-inch × 8-inch baking dish.

Preheat oven to 425°F.

Roll out pie crust to cover the apple mixture.

Place crust on apple mixture.

Cut crust into 1-inch squares.

Bake until juice begins to bubble and apples are tender, about 40 minutes.

Rhubarb Custard Pie

Yield: One 9-inch pie

Custard:

2 Tbs. sugar

2 Tbs. cornstarch

⅛ tsp. salt

1 cup soy milk

1½ tsp. vanilla

Filling:

3 cups ½-inch diced rhubarb

½ cup sugar

1½ Tbs. lemon juice

Crumb Topping:

⅓ cup brown sugar

¼ cup flour

⅓ cup quick cooking oatmeal, uncooked

2 Tbs. vegetable oil

Single Pie Crust (pg. 334)

Custard:

In a 3-quart saucepan, combine ingredients for custard filling. Heat until thickened, stirring constantly. Set aside.

Filling:

In a large bowl, combine filling ingredients and set aside.

Crumb Topping:

In a medium bowl combine crumb topping ingredients and set aside.

Assembling pie:

Preheat oven to 375°F.

Rhubarb Custard Pie
(*continued*)

Prepare pie crust. Line a 9-inch pie dish with the crust.

Pour in custard.

Top custard with rhubarb filling.

Bake for 20 minutes.

Remove pie from oven.

Top with crumb topping.

Return pie to oven and continue to bake for 30 minutes.

Chill before serving.

Southern Style Peach Pie

Yield: One 9-inch pie

6 cups peeled* and sliced fresh peaches (about 8 fresh peaches)

¾ cup sugar

⅓ cup quick tapioca

1/8 tsp. cinnamon (optional)

1 Tbs. lemon juice

9-inch Double Pie Crust (pg. 332)

Preheat oven to 425°F.

In a large bowl combine the peaches, sugar, tapioca, cinnamon, and lemon juice. Let sit for 15 minutes to let tapioca soften.

Prepare pie crust. Line bottom of pie dish with bottom crust.

Pour peach mixture into pie dish.

Cover with top crust and seal edges.

With a dinner knife, pierce the top crust a few times to allow steam to escape.

Bake until juice begins to bubble, about 40 minutes.

** To peel stubborn peaches, place peaches in boiling water for 30-60 seconds. After boiling, immediately place peaches in cold water. The skins should slip right off.*

Strawberry Chocolate Cream Pie

Yield: One pie

1 Graham Cracker Crust (pg. 333) or 1 single precooked Pie Crust (pg. 334)

8 oz. semisweet vegan baking chocolate squares, chopped

14-oz. can unsweetened light coconut milk

1 pint fresh strawberries, stemmed and ¼-inch sliced

Prepare pie crust and set aside.

Place chocolate in a medium bowl and set aside.

In a small saucepan bring coconut milk to a boil.

Pour over chocolate and let sit for five minutes.

Whisk until smooth.

Set aside 8 nice slices of strawberries for topping the pie.

Line bottom of pie crust with remaining strawberries.

Pour chocolate over strawberries.

Top with the 8 reserved strawberries (one per slice).

Chill until set.

Strawberry Rhubarb Pie

Yield: One 9-inch pie

1¼ cups sugar

¼ cup cornstarch

4 cups ½-inch sliced rhubarb

2 cups ½-inch sliced strawberries

9-inch Double Pie Crust (pg. 332)

In a large bowl, combine sugar and cornstarch.

Stir in rhubarb.

Gently stir in strawberries.

Preheat oven to 400°F.

Prepare pie crusts and line bottom of pie dish with bottom crust.

Pour rhubarb mixture into pie dish.

Cover with top crust and seal edges.

With a dinner knife, pierce the top crust a few times to allow steam to escape.

Bake until juice begins to bubble, about 45 minutes.

Tapioca Coconut Pudding

Yield: 3 servings

⅓ cup small pearl tapioca, uncooked

14-oz. can unsweetened coconut milk

¾ cup soy milk

½ cup water

½ cup sugar

2 Tbs. vanilla

In a 3-quart saucepan, combine all ingredients.

Let tapioca soak for 30 minutes.

Place saucepan on stove and bring to a boil, stirring constantly.

Once boiling, reduce heat to low and simmer for 30 minutes, stirring frequently.

Remove from heat, cover and let sit for 10 minutes.

Refrigerate until chilled.

Thai Coconut Lime Bean Pudding

Yield: 4 servings

- **½ cup uncooked adzuki beans, rinsed**
- **¼ cup brown sugar**
- **¾ tsp. cinnamon**
- **¾ tsp. salt**
- **⅓ cup small pearl tapioca**
- **½ cup sugar**
- **14-oz. can unsweetened coconut milk**
- **¾ cup soy milk**
- **½ cup water**
- **1½ tsp. vanilla**
- **¼ tsp. almond extract**
- **Zest of one lime**
- **Juice of one lime**

In a large pot, boil beans until tender, about 1½ hours.

Drain and rinse beans with cold water.

Place beans in a bowl and add brown sugar, cinnamon, and salt. Refrigerate until needed.

In a 3-quart saucepan, combine remaining ingredients.

Let tapioca soak for 30 minutes.

Place saucepan on stove and bring to a boil, stirring constantly.

Once boiling, reduce heat to low and simmer for 30 minutes, stirring frequently.

Remove from heat. Cover and let sit for 10 minutes.

Refrigerate until chilled.

To serve, place ¼ cup of cooked beans in an individual serving dish and top with ½ cup of pudding.

Sauces/Dips/Spreads:

Ancho Sauce

Yield: 2 cups

- **1 cup vegetable broth**
- **2 tomatoes, medium dice**
- **1 dried ancho chili, stemmed and seeds removed**
- **¼ cup small diced onion**
- **¼ cup raisins**
- **¼ tsp. oregano**
- **¼ tsp. cumin**
- **Salt to taste (about 1½ tsp.)**

In a 2-quart saucepan, combine all ingredients except salt.

Bring to a boil.

Reduce heat to low and simmer for 15 minutes, stirring occasionally.

Carefully place in a blender and blend until smooth.

Add salt to taste.

Reheat if needed.

Asian Dipping Sauce

Use this sauce in a stir-fry or as a dipping sauce.

Yield: 1¾ cup

1 cup vegetable broth

⅓ cup brown sugar

¼ cup soy sauce

2 Tbs. cornstarch

In a 2-quart saucepan, whisk together all ingredients.

Heat sauce until hot and thickened, stirring occasionally.

Baba Ganoush

Yield: 2½ cups

2 whole unpeeled eggplants

1½ cups chopped onions

1 cup peeled garlic gloves

½ cup olive oil

¼ cup tahini

¼ cup lemon juice

Salt to taste (about 2 tsp.)

Preheat oven to 425°F.

Bake eggplant until tender, about 20-40 minutes, turning once.

Cut eggplant in half and scoop out eggplant. Set aside.

In a large pan, sauté the onion and garlic with the oil until tender, about 10 minutes.

In a food processor, combine eggplant, onions, garlic, tahini, and lemon juice.

Process until smooth.

Add salt to taste.

Serve chilled

Barbecue Sauce

Yield: 2 cups

6-oz. can tomato paste

½ cup water

¾ cup brown sugar

3 Tbs. apple cider vinegar

3 tsp. salt

1 tsp. liquid smoke

In a 2-quart saucepan, combine all ingredients.

Heat until hot.

Simmer for five minutes.

Brown Mustard Sauce

Great on Reuben sandwiches.

Yield: 1½ cups

1 small onion, minced

2 Tbs. vegetable oil

½ cup prepared brown mustard

½ cup vegan sour cream

In a 2-quart saucepan, sauté the onion with the oil until tender.

Transfer onions to a bowl, add mustard and sour cream and stir until combined.

Caramel Sauce

Yield: 1 cup

¾ cup light brown sugar, packed

1½ tsp. cornstarch

⅓ cup soy milk

1 tsp. vanilla

¼ cup vegan margarine

In a 2-quart saucepan, whisk together the brown sugar, cornstarch, soy milk, and vanilla.

Add margarine.

Heat to a boil, whisking constantly.

Reduce heat to low and simmer for five minutes, stirring occasionally.

Cherry Sauce

Good on ice cream or as a cranberry sauce alternative.

Yield: 1½ cups

1 cup dried and pitted sweet cherries

⅓ cup water

2 Tbs. brown sugar

2 Tbs. sugar

¾ tsp. cornstarch

In a 2-quart saucepan, combine all ingredients.

Bring to a boil, stirring constantly.

Remove from heat and cover for 10 minutes.

If preferred, transfer to a food processor and process until smooth.

Chipotle Dipping Sauce

Yield: about ½ cup

½ cup vegan mayonnaise or vegan sour cream

1 Tbs. Tabasco Chipotle Sauce or favorite hot sauce

Salt to taste (about ¼ tsp.)

In a small bowl, whisk together the mayonnaise or sour cream with the hot sauce.

Add salt to taste.

Coconut Curry Sauce

Yield: 1½ cups

2 Tbs. flour

1 Tbs. curry powder

2 Tbs. vegetable oil

14-oz. can unsweetened coconut milk

1 Tbs. soy sauce

Salt to taste (about ½ tsp.)

In a 2-quart saucepan combine flour, curry powder, and oil.

Heat until it starts to bubble, stirring constantly.

Add coconut milk and soy sauce.

Cook until hot and thickened, stirring constantly.

Add salt to taste.

Thailand

Coconut Peanut Sauce

Serve hot or cold.

Yield: 1½ cups

5.5-oz. can unsweetened coconut milk (¾ cup)

½ cup peanut butter

1 Tbs. soy sauce

1 tsp. sesame oil

½ tsp. salt

Vegan sriracha sauce to taste

In a bowl, combine coconut milk, peanut butter, soy sauce, sesame oil, and salt.

Add sriracha sauce to taste.

Coconut Pumpkin Miso Sauce

Great over rice or tofu.

Yield: 2 cups

14-oz. can unsweetened coconut milk

2 Tbs. pumpkin puree

1 Tbs. cornstarch

1 Tbs. miso paste

In a 2-quart saucepan, whisk together all ingredients.

Heat until hot and thickened, stirring constantly.

Country Gravy

Yield: 3 cups

⅓ cup flour

¼ cup vegetable oil

2½ cups unsweetened soy milk

2 tsp. onion powder

Salt to taste (about 1 tsp.)

Pepper to taste (about ½ tsp.)

In a 2-quart saucepan, combine flour and oil.

Cook until bubbling, stirring constantly.

Add soy milk and onion powder.

Heat until hot and thickened, stirring constantly.

Add salt and pepper to taste.

Dijon Sauce

Yield: 1¼ cups

½ cup small diced onion

2 Tbs. vegetable oil

2 Tbs. flour

⅛ tsp. black pepper

1 Tbs. Dijon mustard

¾ cup unsweetened soy milk

Salt to taste (about 1 tsp.)

In a 2-quart saucepan, sauté the onion with the oil until tender.

Add flour, black pepper, and Dijon mustard. Cook for one minute, stirring constantly.

Add soy milk.

Heat sauce until hot and thickened, stirring constantly.

Add salt to taste.

Edamame Jade Pesto

Yield: 1¾ cups

½ onion, small dice

1 clove garlic, peeled

½ cup olive oil

¼ cup minced ginger

¼ cup rice vinegar

1 cup shelled edamame

1 bunch cilantro, stemmed and chopped

Salt to taste (about 1½ tsp.)

In a 3-quart saucepan, sauté the onion and garlic with the olive oil until caramelized, about 10 minutes.

Add ginger and rice vinegar. Cook for five minutes.

Add edamame and cook for two minutes.

Carefully place mixture in a food processor.

Add cilantro and process until smooth.

Add salt to taste.

Reheat if needed.

Enchilada Sauce

Yield: 2½ cups

2½ tsp. chili powder

1 tsp. sugar

1 tsp. onion powder

2 Tbs. vegetable oil

6-oz. can tomato paste

1¼ cups water

Salt to taste (about ¾ tsp.)

In a 2-quart saucepan, combine chili powder, sugar, onion powder, and oil.

Cook until bubbly, stirring constantly.

Add tomato paste and water.

Bring to a low boil, stirring frequently.

Add salt to taste.

Mexico

Guacamole

A popular shortcut for guacamole is to simply add your favorite salsa to diced avocado.

Yield: 2 cups

2 ripe avocados, peeled and pitted

1 ripe tomato, small dice

¼ cup chopped cilantro

2 Tbs. lemon juice

½ tsp. garlic powder

Salt to taste (about ¼ tsp.)

Dice or mash avocado.

In a small bowl, combine avocado, cilantro, lemon juice, and garlic powder.

Add salt to taste.

Hummus

For a smoother garlic flavor, roast the peeled garlic cloves with the olive oil before processing (see recipe). For a stronger garlic flavor, add garlic powder to taste.

Yield: 1½ cups

15-oz. can garbanzo beans, drained and rinsed

3 Tbs. lemon juice

1 Tbs. tahini*

2 Tbs. olive oil

4 cloves fresh garlic, peeled and crushed, or use Roasted Garlic if desired

Salt to taste (about ½ tsp.)

Place all ingredients except salt in a food processor and process until smooth.

Add salt to taste.

* *Tahini is a traditional ingredient in hummus but may be omitted.*

Roasted Garlic

In a small baking dish, toss peeled garlic with olive oil.

Bake for 20 minutes at 375°F.

Kung Pao Sauce

Yield: 2 cups

½ onion, small dice

2 stalks celery, small dice

1 Tbs. sesame oil

3 Tbs. peanut butter

½ cup soy sauce

½ cup water

¼ cup brown sugar

1 tsp. cornstarch

½ tsp. ginger

⅛ tsp. cayenne pepper

In a 3-quart saucepan, sauté the onion and celery with the oil until tender.

In a bowl, whisk together remaining ingredients.

Add to pan.

Heat until hot and thickened, stirring frequently.

Marinara Sauce

Yield: 4 cups

½ onion, small dice

3 Tbs. olive oil

1 Tbs. basil

2 tsp. onion powder

2 tsp. oregano

1 tsp. sugar

2 Tbs. balsamic vinegar

28-oz. can crushed tomatoes

6-oz. can tomato paste

Salt to taste (about 2 tsp.)

In a 3-quart saucepan, sauté the onion with the oil until tender.

Add the basil, onion powder, oregano, and sugar.

Add vinegar and cook for one minute.

Add crushed tomatoes and tomato paste.

Cover and simmer for 10 minutes, stirring occasionally.

Add salt to taste.

France

Mayonnaise

Refrigerate and use mayonnaise within one week.

Yield: 3 cups

1 cup sweetened or unsweetened soy milk

1 Tbs. apple cider vinegar or distilled vinegar

1 Tbs. sugar

1¼ tsp. salt

¾ tsp. dry mustard

2 cups vegetable oil

In a food processor, process the soy milk, vinegar, sugar, salt, and dry mustard for one minute.

With food processor running, slowly stream in oil.

After all the oil has been added, continue to run food processor for one minute.

Chill mayonnaise until set, about two hours.

Keep refrigerated.

Mole Sauce

Yield: 2 cups

1 cup vegetable broth

2 small tomatoes, medium dice

1 dried ancho chili, stemmed and seeds removed

½ cup medium diced onion

¼ cup raisins

2 Tbs. sugar

¼ tsp. oregano

¼ tsp. cumin

1 oz. unsweetened baking chocolate, chopped

Salt to taste (about 1½ tsp.)

In a 2-quart saucepan, combine all ingredients except chocolate and salt.

Bring to a boil.

Reduce heat to low and simmer for 15 minutes, stirring occasionally.

In a blender, add simmered ingredients and chocolate. Blend until smooth.

Add salt to taste.

Reheat if needed.

Pad Thai Sauce

Yield: 2½ cups

⅔ cup lime juice (about 6 limes)

½ cup soy sauce

⅓ cup seasoned rice vinegar

¾ cup sugar

2 Tbs. tamarind paste (optional)

Vegan sriracha sauce to taste, about 2 Tbs. (optional)

In a bowl, whisk together the lime juice, soy sauce, rice vinegar, sugar, and tamarind paste.

Add vegan sriracha sauce to taste.

Peanut Sauce

Yield: 1 cup

½ cup unsweetened peanut butter

¼ cup sesame oil

2 Tbs. soy sauce

2 Tbs. water

⅛ tsp. cayenne pepper

In a small bowl, combine all ingredients.

Pesto Sauce

To help keep the pesto from turning brown: Use cold ingredients and minimize the food processing time for the basil, stir prepared pesto sauce into cooked hot pasta just before serving, and store leftovers in an airtight container.

Yield: 1 cup

15 peeled cloves of garlic (one whole garlic bulb)

½ cup olive oil

¼ cup pine nuts or walnuts

¾ tsp. salt

2 bunches basil, stemmed

Preheat oven to 375°F.

In a small baking dish, toss garlic with olive oil.

Bake for 20 minutes.

Cool garlic with its roasting oil in the refrigerator for 30 minutes.

In a food processor, combine roasted garlic, roasting oil, pine nuts or walnuts, and salt until smooth.

Add basil and pulse blade just until smooth.

Pico De Gallo

For a gourmet touch, use one red tomato and one yellow tomato.

Yield: 4 cups

2 tomatoes, small dice

½ onion, small dice

½ cup chopped cilantro

¼ cup lemon juice (about 1 lemon)

1 jalapeño, chopped (optional)

Salt to taste (about ½ tsp.)

In a small bowl, combine tomatoes, onion, cilantro, lemon juice, and jalapeño.

Add salt to taste.

Chill before serving.

Pizza Sauce

Yield: 1 cup (Enough for 1 large pizza, 2 medium pizzas, or 6 calzones)

6 oz. tomato paste

1 tsp. basil

1 tsp. oregano

½ tsp. garlic powder

½ tsp. onion powder

¾ tsp. salt

2 Tbs. water

1 Tbs. olive oil

In a small bowl, whisk together all ingredients.

Plum Sauce

Yield: 2 cups

6 plums, pitted and quartered

½ cup brown sugar

¼ cup water

3 Tbs. chopped fresh ginger

3 Tbs. soy sauce

3 Tbs. lemon juice

2 Tbs. cornstarch

In a blender, blend all ingredients until smooth.

Transfer to a 2-quart saucepan.

Heat until hot and thickened, stirring constantly.

Raita

Yield: 2 cups

1 cucumber, peeled and seeds removed

12 oz. vegan plain yogurt or vegan sour cream (1½ cups)

½ bunch mint, stemmed, minced (optional)

3 Tbs. lemon juice

1 tsp. garlic powder

½ tsp. cumin

¼ tsp. cayenne pepper (optional)

Salt to taste (about ½ tsp.)

Shred or small dice (diced cucumber is traditional but I prefer shredded) cucumber into a medium-sized bowl.

Add yogurt or sour cream, mint, lemon juice, garlic powder, cumin, and cayenne.

Add salt to taste.

Spicy Orange Sauce

Yield: 2 cups

1 cup frozen unsweetened orange juice concentrate

1 cup water

⅓ cup sugar

¼ cup soy sauce

1 Tbs. rice vinegar

3 Tbs. cornstarch

¼ tsp. cayenne pepper or ½ tsp. crushed red pepper flakes

In a 3-quart saucepan, whisk together all ingredients.

Heat until hot and thickened, stirring frequently.

Sweet and Sour Sauce, version 1

Yield: 2½ cups

½ onion, medium dice

1 red bell pepper, medium dice

2 Tbs. fresh minced ginger (optional)

2 Tbs. vegetable oil

4-oz. can pineapple chunks or tidbits with liquid

¼ cup soy sauce

¼ cup rice vinegar

½ cup cold water, divided

¼ cup sugar

2 Tbs. lemon juice

1½ Tbs. cornstarch

In a 3-quart saucepan, sauté the onion, pepper, and ginger with the oil until tender.

Add pineapple with its liquid, soy sauce, vinegar, ¼ cup of the cold water, sugar, and lemon juice. Heat until boiling.

In a small bowl, whisk together the cornstarch and the remaining ¼ cup of cold water.

Slowly stream cornstarch slurry into sauce while whisking constantly.

Heat until hot and thickened.

Sweet and Sour Sauce, version 2

Yield: 1⅓ cups

½ cup rice vinegar

½ cup soy sauce

¼ cup water

2 Tbs. cornstarch

¾ cup brown sugar

In a 3-quart saucepan, whisk together all ingredients.

Heat until hot and thickened, stirring constantly.

Sweet Chili Sauce

Yield: 1¼ cups

¼ cup lime juice

¼ cup lemon juice

¼ cup soy sauce

¼ cup vegan sweet chili sauce

¼ cup brown sugar

¼ cup sugar

In a mixing bowl, whisk together all ingredients.

Tapenade

Yield: 2 cups

7 peeled garlic cloves

¼ cup olive oil

1 cup pitted Kalamata olives

¼ cup capers, drained and rinsed

½ bunch fresh basil, stems removed

Preheat oven to 375°F.

In a small baking dish, toss garlic with olive oil.

Bake for 20 minutes.

Cool garlic and oil for 30 minutes in refrigerator.

In a food processor, combine garlic, olive oil, olives, capers, and basil.

Process until nearly smooth.

Thai Coconut Sauce

Serve over rice, noodles, vegetables, or tofu.

Yield: 2 cups

2 Tbs. vegetable oil

2 Tbs. flour

1½ Tbs. vegan yellow curry paste

14-oz. can unsweetened coconut milk

1 Tbs. soy sauce

In a 2-quart saucepan, combine oil, flour, and curry paste. Cook on low heat for one minute, stirring constantly.

Add coconut milk and soy sauce.

Heat on medium heat until hot and thickened, stirring constantly.

Thai Pumpkin Coconut Sauce

Yield: 3 cups

1 Tbs. curry powder

1 Tbs. vegetable oil

1 cup pumpkin puree

14-oz. can unsweetened coconut milk

2 Tbs. soy sauce

Salt to taste (about ½ tsp.)

In a 3-quart saucepan, combine curry powder and oil.

Cook until lightly bubbling.

Add pumpkin, coconut milk, and soy sauce.

Heat on medium heat until hot and thickened.

Add salt to taste.

Tomatillo Sauce

Yield: 3 cups

1 lb. tomatillos (6 large), husks removed

½ onion, small dice

2 Tbs. vegetable oil

1 tsp. onion powder

7-oz. can diced green chilies

2 Tbs. lemon juice

Salt to taste (about 1 tsp.)

Boil tomatillos just until tender, about 20 minutes. Drain off water and set aside.

In a 2-quart saucepan, sauté the onion with the oil until tender.

In a blender, blend the cooked tomatillos, sautéed onion, onion powder, diced green chilies, and lemon juice.

Return to saucepan and heat until hot.

Add salt to taste.

Tzatziki Sauce

Tzatziki sauce is the traditional dressing served with falafel and gyros.

Yield: 1 cup

½ cucumber, peeled and ends removed

¾ cup vegan plain yogurt or vegan sour cream

1½ Tbs. lemon juice

½ tsp. garlic powder

Salt to taste (about ¼ tsp.)

Shred or small dice (diced cucumber is traditional but I prefer shredded) cucumber into a medium-sized bowl.

Add the yogurt or sour cream, lemon juice, and garlic.

Add salt to taste.

England

Worcestershire Sauce

Yield: ½ cup

1 cup apple cider vinegar

¼ cup soy sauce

2 Tbs. brown sugar

1 Tbs. tamarind paste or 2 Tbs. raisins

½ tsp. garlic powder

½ tsp. onion powder

½ tsp. dry mustard

¼ tsp. black pepper

⅛ tsp. cinnamon

In a saucepan, combine all ingredients.

Bring to a boil, stir frequently, and reduce sauce down to ½ cup.

If using raisins, blend until smooth.

Chill.

Supporting Recipes:

Almond Glaze

Yield: 1½ cups

2 cups powdered sugar

¼ cup water

¾ tsp. almond extract

⅓ cup vegan margarine

In a saucepan, whisk together the powdered sugar, water, and almond extract.

Add margarine.

Place on stove and bring to a boil.

Remove from heat and cool slightly before using.

Basic Dough

2¼ cups flour*

2 tsp. salt

3 Tbs. olive oil

¾ cup warm water

** Use part whole wheat if preferred (add 2 Tbs. water for every one cup of whole wheat flour used).*

In a large bowl, combine flour and salt.

Stir in oil and water.

On a floured surface, knead dough for five minutes.

Cover and let rest until needed.

Cajun Seasoning

Yield: ¼ cup

2 Tbs. paprika

2 tsp. garlic powder

2 tsp. salt

1 tsp. onion powder

1 tsp. cayenne pepper

In a small bowl, combine all ingredients.

Chocolate Glaze

Yield: 1¾ cups

⅓ cup vegan margarine

¼ cup cocoa powder

1 Tbs. vanilla

¼ cup water

2 cups powdered sugar

In a small saucepan, heat margarine until melted.

Whisk in cocoa powder.

Add vanilla and water.

Remove from heat and whisk in powdered sugar.

Cream Cheese Frosting

Yield: Will frost a double-layer 8-inch cake

½ cup vegan cream cheese

½ cup vegan margarine

2 cups powdered sugar

With an electric mixer, beat all ingredients just until smooth.

Refrigerate 30 minutes before using if necessary to help set frosting.

Croutons

Yield: 6 cups

8 slices of bread, cubed

3 Tbs. olive oil

1½ tsp. basil

1½ tsp. onion powder

1 tsp. oregano

1 tsp. paprika

¾ tsp. salt

Preheat oven to 375°F.

In a large baking dish, toss together all ingredients.

Bake until bread is crisp (about 20 minutes), stirring every five minutes.

After completely cooled, store in an airtight container.

Drop Biscuits

Yield: 12

3½ cups flour*

5 tsp. baking powder

1½ tsp. salt

1½ cups soy milk

⅔ cup vegetable oil

** Use part whole wheat flour if you prefer.*

Preheat oven to 425°F.

In a large bowl, whisk together the flour, baking powder, and salt.

With a spoon, stir in the soy milk and oil just until combined.

Scoop or spoon biscuits onto a lightly oiled baking sheet.

Bake until done, about 14 minutes.

Hot Fudge Sauce

Yield: 1½ cups

1 cup sugar

3 Tbs. cocoa powder

4 tsp. cornstarch

⅛ tsp. salt

1 cup soy milk

1 tsp. vanilla

In a 2-quart saucepan, whisk together the sugar, cocoa powder, cornstarch, and salt.

Whisk in the soy milk.

Heat until boiling, stirring constantly.

Remove from heat and stir in vanilla.

Cool to desired temperature before serving.

Maple Frosting

Yield: Enough to frost 20 doughnuts

1¾ cups powdered sugar

2 Tbs. water

2 tsp. maple extract

¼ cup vegan margarine

In a saucepan, whisk together the powdered sugar, water, and maple extract.

Add margarine.

Place on stove and bring to a boil, stirring frequently.

Remove from heat and cool slightly before using.

Meatballs

Yield: 24 meatballs

1¼ cups vital wheat gluten flour

1 Tbs. paprika

1½ tsp. onion powder

1½ tsp. garlic powder

1½ tsp. basil

1½ tsp. oregano

¼ tsp. ground black pepper

1½ tsp. salt

¾ cup water

½ cup vegetable oil, divided

In a large bowl, whisk together the dry ingredients.

Add water and ¼ cup of the oil all at once and stir until well combined.

Form dough into walnut-sized balls.

Place a steamer basket in the bottom of a large pan. Add water to just below the steamer basket. Bring water to a boil. Place meatballs in basket leaving ½ inch between meatballs (cook in batches if needed).

Cover pan with tight-fitting lid and steam meatballs until done, about 15 minutes.

Place meatballs in a colander to drain.

In a large frying pan, sauté the meatballs with the remaining ¼ cup of oil until browned.

Parmesan Cheese

Sprinkle on top of pasta, salads, or soups.

Yield: 2 cups

2 cups slivered or sliced almonds

¼ cup nutritional yeast flakes

¼ cup basil

2 Tbs. onion powder

1 Tbs. garlic powder

1 Tbs. oregano

1 Tbs. dried lemon peel

1 tsp. salt

½ tsp. paprika

¼ tsp. nutmeg

Place all ingredients in a food processor and process to cornmeal consistency.

Store in a sealed container in the refrigerator.

Pasta, homemade

Yield: 4 servings

1½ cups semolina flour*

½ tsp. salt

½ cup water

1 Tbs. vegetable oil

** Use part whole wheat flour if you prefer. Additional water may be needed.*

In a bowl, whisk together the flour and salt.

Stir in the water and oil.

On a non-floured surface, knead dough for 10 minutes.

Cover dough and let rest for 10 minutes.

Divided dough into two pieces.

On a lightly floured surface, roll out each piece to ⅛-inch thick.

Cut pasta into desired shapes.

Let pasta dry on a lightly floured surface for a minimum of one hour.

Bring a large pot of water to a boil. Add pasta and stir constantly the first minute and occasionally afterwards until the pasta is done, about five minutes.

Pie Crust, double

Yield: Makes two single-layer pie crusts, or one top and one bottom pie crust.

2⅔ cups flour*

1½ tsp. salt

¾ cup vegetable oil

¼ cup cold water

** Part Whole Wheat Pie Crust: Substitute one cup of flour with one cup of whole wheat flour and add additional water as needed.*

In a large bowl, thoroughly mix the flour and salt.

Stir in the oil and water with a dinner fork just until combined (do not overwork pastry).

Divide dough into two balls. Roll each ball between two pieces of waxed paper or on a lightly floured surface to desired size.

Precooked bottom pie crust:

Pierce bottom and sides of crust with a fork. Cook in a 425°F oven for 13 minutes.

Pie Crust, graham cracker

Yield: One 9-inch pie crust

10 vegan graham crackers

¼ cup vegan margarine, softened

3 Tbs. sugar

If you have a food processor:

Grind crackers in food processor to fine crumbs.

Add margarine and sugar and blend until combined.

Press crumbs into the bottom of the pie dish and up the sides.

Chill in refrigerator before filling.

If you don't have a food processor:

Place crackers in a plastic bag and crush with a rolling pin.

Pour crumbs into a large bowl.

Stir in margarine and sugar until well combined.

Press crumbs into the bottom of the dish and up the sides.

Chill in refrigerator before filling.

Pie Crust, single

Yield: One single-layer 9-inch pie crust

1¾ cups flour*

1 tsp. salt

½ cup vegetable oil

3 Tbs. cold water

* *Whole Wheat Pie Crust: Substitute ½ cup of flour with ½ cup of whole wheat flour and add additional water as needed.*

In a large bowl, thoroughly mix the flour and salt.

Stir in the oil and water with a dinner fork just until combined (do not overwork pastry).

Roll dough out between two pieces of waxed paper or on a lightly floured surface to desired size.

Precooked Pie Crust:

Pierce bottom and sides of crust with a fork. Cook in a 425°F oven for 13 minutes.

Quinoa

Yield: 3 cups

1 cup quinoa, rinsed

1½ cups water

In a 3-quart saucepan, bring quinoa and water to a boil.

Reduce heat to low, cover, and simmer until quinoa is tender and all water is absorbed, about 18-20 minutes (additional water may be added during the cooking process if you prefer a tenderer quinoa).

Ricotta Cheese

Yield: 2½ cups

20 oz. vegan mozzarella or jack cheese, medium dice

2 Tbs. lemon juice

1 tsp. salt

In a food processor, process all ingredients until smooth.

Roasted Edamame

Yield: 1½ cups

8 oz. frozen shelled edamame (2 cups)

2 Tbs. soy sauce

1 Tbs. minced fresh ginger

1 Tbs. vegetable oil

Preheat oven to 350°F.

In a 9-inch × 13-inch baking dish, toss all ingredients.

Bake, stirring every 10 minutes, until lightly crisp on the outside and tender on the inside, about 40 minutes.

Tempura Batter

Yield: 2 cups

1¼ cups flour

¼ cup cornstarch

1 Tbs. salt

2 tsp. baking powder

1¼ cups soy milk

In a large shallow bowl, whisk together the dry ingredients.

Whisk in the soy milk.

Roasted Marinated Tofu

Serve with rice or chilled in a salad or sandwich.

Yield: 4 servings

16 oz. extra firm tofu

¼ cup lemon juice

¼ cup lime juice

¼ cup soy sauce

½ cup brown sugar

Preheat oven to 375°F.

Cut tofu into four slabs and place in a 9-inch × 13-inch baking dish.

In a bowl, combine remaining ingredients.

Pour over tofu.

Bake for 45 minutes.

Chill if preferred.

Variation: Roasted Thai Marinated Tofu

Add 2 Tbs. vegan sriracha sauce to marinade.

Vanilla Glaze

Yield: 1½ cups

2 cups powdered sugar

¼ cup water

1 Tbs. vanilla

⅓ cup vegan margarine

In a saucepan, whisk together the powdered sugar, water, and vanilla extract.

Add margarine.

Place on stove and bring to a boil.

Remove from heat and cool slightly before using.

Whipped Cream

Yield: 2 cups

2 14-oz. cans unsweetened and regular fat coconut milk, chilled overnight

½ cup powdered sugar (optional)

Place coconut milk in refrigerator overnight, right-side up. Do not shake.

Place mixing bowl and electric beaters in freezer for at least 30 minutes before use to chill if the temperature of the room is above 75°F.

Pierce bottom of coconut milk cans with a pointed can opener and drain off the liquid part (leaving thick coconut cream in can).

Open top of coconut milk cans and spoon the coconut cream into the chilled bowl.

Whip coconut cream with chilled beaters until fluffy, about one minute.

Gently whip in powdered sugar.

Keep refrigerated until ready to use.

Will keep in the refrigerator for four days.

Wonton Wrappers

Yield: Sixteen 4-inch round wrappers

1½ cups flour

3 Tbs. vital wheat gluten flour

½ tsp. salt

½ cup warm water

In a medium bowl, whisk together the dry ingredients.

Stir in water.

On an un-floured surface, knead dough for five minutes.

Cover dough and let rest for 20 minutes.

Roll into an 8-inch log.

Cut into 16 pieces.

Roll each piece into a 4-inch circle.

Use as needed.

Cook's Notes:

Be sure to wash all produce before using.

When a recipe calls for flour, use all-purpose white flour unless otherwise noted.

These recipes were made with table salt. If using kosher salt, you may need to increase the salt.

All herbs and spices are dry unless otherwise noted.

Glossary:

Active dry yeast: A leavening agent used in baking.

Blend: To thoroughly mix.

Bulgur: Toasted cracked wheat.

Chill: To cool in a refrigerator until cold.

Chop: To cut into pieces with no consistent size or shape needed.

Couscous: Pasta, smaller than rice, made of semolina from durum wheat flour.

Cream: To thoroughly mix ingredients with a mixer, food processor, or several strokes with a wooden spoon.

Dice: To cut into ¼-inch × ¼-inch pieces. "Large dice" refers to foods cut into ½-inch × ½-inch pieces. "Small dice" refers to foods cut into ⅛-inch × ⅛-inch pieces.

Double boiler: A cooking utensil consisting of two pots that fit one on top of the other. Food is placed in the upper pot and water is boiled in the lower pot. Double boilers are used when food items should not be placed directly on heat.

Egg replacer powder: Made by Ener-G Foods. This is a powder that is used to help foods rise. Not to be confused with liquid egg substitute.

Flours:

AP (all purpose) flour
Medium gluten flour that can be used in most recipes.

bread flour
High gluten flour that is best for breads and pizza dough.

cake flour
Low gluten flour that is best for

cakes, muffins, and quick breads. Same as Pastry Flour.

pastry flour
Low gluten flour that is best for cakes, muffins, and quick breads. Same as cake flour.

vital wheat gluten flour
The naturally occurring protein in wheat. Can be found in packages or sold in bulk.

Garbanzo beans: Also known as chickpeas.

Jalapeño: A finger sized green or red chili that is popular in salsas. It can be found canned or fresh. It has a Scoville unit rating of 25,000.

Julienne: To cut into ¼-inch strips.

Knead: The process of pressing and folding dough until smooth and elastic. Kneading strengthens gluten strands so they can hold in the gas bubbles better.

Marinate: To soak an item in a savory sauce, called a marinade, to add flavor.

Mince: To cut into very small pieces.

Miso: Fermented soybean paste. Sold refrigerated.

Nutritional yeast flakes: An inactive yeast that has no leavening agent and has a cheesy flavor. High in B vitamins and protein.

Polenta: Coarsely ground cornmeal. Also know as grits.

Puree: To process a food with a blender or food processor until smooth.

Roast: To cook in an oven, usually at a high temperature of 375 degrees or hotter.

Sauté: Rapid cooking done in an open pan on medium-high to high heat using minimal oil.

Semolina flour: Flour made from durum wheat. It is high in gluten and protein.

Sesame butter: Another name for tahini. Made from ground sesame seeds.

Shred: To cut into thin short strips. Usually done with a box grater or food processor with a grater attachment.

Simmer: To cook at a low temperature in order to allow ingredient flavors to blend.

Tahini: Also called sesame butter. Made from ground sesame seeds.

Toast: To brown in an oven or in a dry skillet.

Tofu, firm: A firm textured tofu used for dicing, pressing, marinating, grilling, and roasting. Sold packed in water.

Tofu, silken: A very smooth tofu used in baking and beverages. Available in both a water pack and aseptic packaging.

Whisk: To mix ingredients using a wire whip called a whisk.

Zest: The very outer rind of any citrus fruit, not including the inner white of the rind. Zest can be removed with a sharp knife, grater, or zester.

Conversion Charts:

Measurements:

1 tsp. = 5 ml.	¼ cup = 60 ml.	⅔ cup = 160 ml.
3 tsp. = 15 ml.	⅓ cup = 80 ml.	¾ cup = 180 ml.
1 Tbs. = 15 ml.	½ cup = 120 ml.	1 cup = 240 ml.

Weights:

1 oz. = 28 grams	15 oz. = 425 grams	28 oz. = 794 grams

Oven Temperatures:

222°F = 110°C	325°F = 170°C	425°F = 220°C
250°F = 130°C	350°F = 180°C	450°F = 230°C
275°F = 140°C	375°F = 190°C	475°F = 240°C
300°F = 150°C	400°F = 200°C	

Measurement conversions:

3 teaspoons = 1 tablespoon

6 teaspoons = 2 tablespoons = ⅛ cup

8 tablespoons = ½ cup

16 tablespoons = 1 cup

1 cup = ½ pint

2 cups = 1 pint

4 cups = 2 pints = 1 quart

8 cups = 4 pints = 2 quarts = ½ gallon

16 cups = 8 pints = 4 quarts = 1 gallon

Liquid volume conversions:

½ liquid ounce = 1 tablespoon

1 liquid ounce = ⅛ cup

2 liquid ounces = ¼ cup

4 liquid ounces = ½ cup

6 liquid ounces = ¾ cup

8 liquid ounces = 1 cup

16 liquid ounces = 1 pint

32 liquid ounces = 1 quart

64 liquid ounces = ½ gallon

128 liquid ounces = 1 gallon

Abbreviations:

Teaspoon = tsp.

Tablespoon = Tbs.

Ounce = oz.

Fluid ounce = fl. oz.

Pint = pt.

Quart = qt.

Gallon = gal.

Protein List:

Raw nuts & seeds (¼ cup, shelled)

Almonds 7g

Brazil nuts 5g

Cashews 4g

Coconut (shredded) 2g

Filberts/hazelnuts 5g

Flax seeds 5g

Macadamia nuts 2g

Peanuts .8g

Pecans 2g

Pine nuts 4g

Pistachio nuts 6g

Pumpkin seeds 7g

Sesame seeds 7g

Soy nuts. 10g

Sunflower seeds 8g

Walnuts .5g

Beans (1cup of cooked beans)

Adzuki beans. 17g

Black beans 15g

Black-eyed peas 14g

Cannellini 17g

Cranberry beans 17g

Fava beans 13g

Garbanzos (chickpeas). 15g

Great northern beans 15g

Green peas (whole) 9g

Kidney beans. 15g

Lentils .18g

Lima beans 15g

Mung beans 14g

Navy beans 16g

Pinto beans 12g

Soybeans. 29g

Split peas. 16g

Soy products

Tofu, firm (3 oz.). 7–12g

Tofu, extra firm (3 oz.) 7–12g

Tofu, silken (3 oz.) 4–6g

Tempeh (4 oz.). 12–20g

Textured vegetable protein
(¼ cup). 10–12g

Grains (¼ cup cooked)

Amaranth. 7g

Barley, pearled 4–5g

Buckwheat goats. 5–6g

Cornmeal (fine ground) 3g

Cornmeal (polenta, coarse). 3g

Millet, hulled 8.4g

Oat, bran 7g

Quinoa. .5g

Rice, brown 3–5g

Rice, white. 4g

Rice, wild 7g

Spelt, berries 6g

Wheat, whole berries 6–9g

Wheat, bulgur 5–6g

Nut/Seed butters (2 Tbs.)

Almond 5–8g

Cashew 4–5g

Peanut 5–6g

Sesame (tahini) 6g

Soy nut 6–7g

Milk substitutes (1 cup)

Almond 1–2g

Soy, regular 6–9g

Soy, low/nonfat 4g

Rice 1g

Multigrain 5g

Oat 4g

Miscellaneous foods

Farina (¼ cup dry) 5g

Flour, rye (¼ cup). 4g

Flour, white unbleached
(¼ cup). 4g

Flour, whole wheat (¼ cup) 5g

Kamut (¼ cup, cooked) 5g

Kashi (½ cup, cooked) 6g

Oatmeal, quick (½ cup dry) 6g

Popcorn, yellow (¼ cup, kernels) 4g

Vital wheat gluten flour (¼ cup) 21g

Yeast flakes, nutritional (3 Tbs.) 8g

Yeast powder, nutritional (3 tsp.) 8g

Fresh vegetables*

Artichoke (medium) 4g

Asparagus (5 spears) 2g

Beans, string (1 cup) 2g

Beets (½ cup) 1g

Broccoli (½ cup) 2g

Brussels sprouts (½ cup) 2g

Cabbage (½ cup) 1g

Carrots (½ cup) 1g

Cauliflower (½ cup) 1g

Celery (1 cup) 1g

Chard, Swiss (1cup) 3g

Collards (1 cup) 4g

Corn, sweet (1 large cob) 5g

Cucumber* (1 cup) 1g

Eggplant (1 cup) 1g

Fennel (1 medium bulb) 3g

Kale (1 cup) 2.5g

Kohlrabi (1 cup) 3g

Leeks (1 cup) 1g

Lettuce* (1 cup) 1g

Okra (1 cup) 1g

Onion (½ cup) 1g

Parsnip (½ cup) 1g

Peas (½ cup) 4g

Peppers, bell (½ cup) 1g

Potato, baked (2.3 x 4.75-inch) 5g

Radish* (1 cup) 1g

Rhubarb (1 cup) 1g

Rutabaga (1 cup) 2g

Spinach* (1 cup) 1g

Squash, summer (1 cup) 2g

Sweet potato (1 cup) 3g

** All amounts refer to cooked vegetables except starred items, which are uncooked/fresh.*

Index

About the Author

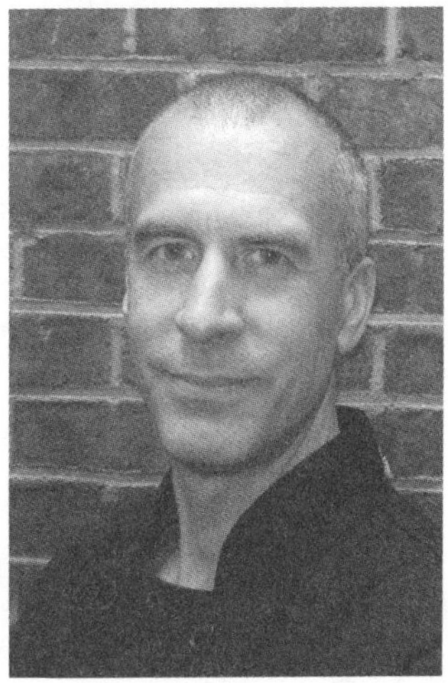

CHEF BRIAN P. McCARTHY has been a professional cook since 1982. In 1995 he turned to a vegan diet for its health benefits, and began to explore the world of vegan cooking as a chef. In Oregon, he ran the Intel vegetarian/vegan international station and prepared dishes for catered events attended by CEOs, mayors, house representatives, senators, and the newly elected Barack Obama. In 2012 Chef McCarthy moved to Massachusetts to cook for the Bon Appétit Management Company, and became an instructor for The Cambridge School of Culinary Arts. He is the author of *The Lantern Vegan Family Cookbook*, and has contributed cooking videos to Everyday Dish.

brianpmccarthy.blogspot.com

About the Publisher

LANTERN BOOKS is dedicated to the principle of living with a greater depth and commitment to the preservation of the natural world. In addition to publishing books on animal advocacy, the environment, health, religion, social justice, and vegetarianism, Lantern prints on recycled paper in the U.S. and saves resources in day-to-day operations. Lantern is honored to be a recipient of the highest standard in environmentally responsible publishing from the Green Press Initiative.

www.lanternbooks.com

Lantern Books has elected to print this title on Natures, a 30% post-consumer recycled paper, processed chlorine-free. As a result, we have saved the following resources:

11 trees, 504 lbs of solid waste, 4559 gallons of water
8 million BTUs, and 993 lbs of greenhouse gases

As part of Lantern Books' commitment to the environment we have joined the Green Press Initiative, a non-profit organization supporting publishers in using fiber that is not sourced from ancient or endangered forests. We hope that you, the reader, will support Lantern and GPI in our endeavor to preserve the ancient forests and the natural systems on which all life depends. One way is to buy books that cost a little more but make a positive commitment to the environment not only in their words, but in the paper that they are printed on. For more information, visit greenpressinitiative.org.